Extend Your Life

Katherine Wright

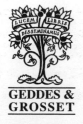

GEDDES &
GROSSET

Published 2002 by Geddes & Grosset,
David Dale House, New Lanark, ML11 9DJ, Scotland

© 2002 Geddes & Grosset

Text by Katherine Wright

First printed 2002
Reprinted 2002

ISBN 1 84205 156 3

Printed and bound in the UK

Contents

Introduction

The advent of the year 2000 was the cause of great celebration throughout the world, but the euphoria has since been replaced by the growing realisation that the planet and its citizens face enormous challenges, as well as great opportunities, in the years that lie ahead. In spite of continuing efforts, the gulf between the rich and poor countries of the world remains wide. A combination of human greed, belligerence and inadequacy, and the occurrence of natural disasters condemns many people to a harsh and frequently short existence.

It is now a certainty that the effects of global warming and climate change will alter the face of the planet and have profound and unpredictable consequences both for its human inhabitants and for animals and plants. The changes will affect the places where people can live, the food that they can grow and eat and the diseases to which they are exposed. It seems likely that the wealthy nations, while not escaping the effects of climate change, will be better placed to try and offset them. However, without very radical changes, the struggle for daily survival seems likely to remain the main priority for the world's most disadvantaged citizens and the effects of global warming will be felt most keenly in the countries where they live.

In Western countries, life has changed dramatically in the last half century since the end of the Second World War and most of the changes have resulted in huge improvements in the quality of human life. The majority of people in Western countries have long since moved beyond the struggle for the basic provision of food, water, shelter and clothing. They enjoy a high standard of living, have access to an enormous variety of foodstuffs from all over the world and benefit from advanced medical and health care. Increased wealth and leisure time mean that most Western people have access to computers, the Internet and other advanced technology and are readily able to become well-informed about matters that affect and interest them.

Advances in medicine and science already mean that successful treatments are now being used against some of the major killer diseases of the past. Some of the conditions and illnesses that are being treated are associated with ageing. In many cases, these treatments are able to restore a quality of life and health that was simply unavailable to people in earlier generations. Other developments in medical science, especially in the field of genetics, have raised the possibility of eliminating some serious disorders altogether while others are aimed at directly tackling the ageing process itself and slowing down its progression. A few scientists have even gone as far as to predict that future research will eventually enable ageing to be 'written out' of the human genome altogether! Of course, people have always been interested in leading a long, healthy and active life but in the past, the means of doing so was often beyond individual control and governed entirely by circumstances. Now, new medical developments and scientific breakthroughs, that are usually widely reported and discussed in the media, are factors that have raised the level of interest in the subject of longevity and achieving a healthy and active old age. People in the West have come to expect that when these advances become available they will have access to them and directly benefit from them.

A second important factor in recent years has been the enormous growth of interest in so-called 'alternative' therapies and philosophies. Most of these claim to promote good health and longevity by giving advice on essential aspects of life such as diet, exercise and lifestyle management, and ways of preventing disease. Both disease prevention and treatment of ailments are based upon natural remedies, usually derived from plants and herbs. However, alternative philosophies are even more wide-ranging, being concerned with the emotional and spiritual aspects of life in addition to dealing with the body and physical factors. Conventional medicine used to be almost exclusively concerned with the treatment of disease and this obviously remains its most important function. However, in recent years, the medical profession as a whole has become far more involved with disease prevention and with the essential factors listed above, i.e. diet, the need for exercise and management of modern lifestyles. These factors, especially diet and nutrition, have become industries in themselves and ones in which the desire to make large profits at times conflicts with more altruistic motives!

The purpose of this book is to attempt to draw all these threads together. It is hoped that ways in which an ordinary person can influence his or her own life span and health will be discovered, by examining the essential aspects of life, both physical, emotional and spiritual, and looking at the advice offered by medicine, science and alternative therapies. New developments and their implications for individual people are looked at and discussed. Some of the more controversial 'treatments' for ageing such as hormonal anti-ageing programmes are included, and their potential dangers as well as possible benefits are examined.

Modern Living

A COMPARISON of life in the early 20th and 21st centuries shows just how greatly human life expectancy and health have improved overall in the last 100 years. How does life in Britain at the start of the 21st century compare with that of 100 years ago?

Life in the early 20th century
In the first half of the 20th century there were no antibiotics and vaccination was still in its infancy. Slum dwellings in the major cities of Britain were still commonplace and many people lived in overcrowded and unhealthy conditions. In these circumstances, infectious diseases were readily able to spread, carrying off both adults and children alike. An example of this was the Spanish 'flu epidemic that killed 228,000 people in Britain between the years 1918 to 1919 and millions more worldwide. Complications resulting from influenza, such as pneumonia, are still a cause of death among the elderly, ill and vulnerable, but protective vaccination and good health care mean that most people survive.

Both maternal and infant mortality were higher

during the early years of the 20th century. Fewer births took place in hospital and advanced medical and surgical techniques were not, in any case, available. This meant that childbirth was a far more hazardous event for women than is the case today when maternal deaths are very rare. Sadly, even the advanced obstetric and neonatal care that is available in modern maternity units cannot prevent the loss of some babies at, or soon after, birth. However, it is certain that many more of these infants are saved, including some that are very premature or born with serious, life-threatening conditions, than were in the past. Hence, although the process of birth remains one of the most dangerous periods in any woman's life, it is safer in the 21st century than at any time previously!

Babies and young children are vulnerable to infections because they have an immature immune system. In the early 1900s, many children were left damaged or even died from common infectious diseases such as scarlet fever, poliomyelitis, diphtheria, measles and smallpox. A combination of vaccination and antibiotics effectively protects the children of today against these formerly dreaded diseases and smallpox has apparently been eradicated completely.

The 1940s and '50s
The development of antibiotics in the 1940s and '50s marked a turning point in modern medicine, enabling

deadly infections to be treated effectively for the first time. Although antibiotic resistance among disease-causing microorganisms has since become a worrying problem, especially in hospitals, antibiotics continue to save many lives.

In the early 20th century, industrial and domestic processes were heavily reliant upon coal as the major source of fuel. Air quality in the larger cities was often poor and some, including London, were regularly affected by choking smog. Respiratory and other industrial illnesses were commonplace and resulted from dirty working conditions and polluted air. These illnesses were a major cause of disability and premature death and although the dangers were recognized, it took many years for the situation to improve through the implementation of 'clean air' Acts and measures to protect people in their place of work. In 21st century Britain, the dirty air from the old, heavy industries is a thing of the past but it has been replaced by new, invisible hazards.

21st-century hazards

Emissions from vehicle exhausts have introduced other forms of pollution, and air quality is still often poor. It is thought that modern air pollution is still a cause of premature death and of disabling illnesses such as bronchitis and asthma. Also, the burning of fossil fuels and particularly the emissions from vehicle exhausts are blamed for the large holes that have appeared in the ozone layer of the atmosphere that screens the Earth from harmful ultraviolet (UV) radiation. The increased amount of UV radiation reaching the planet's surface is responsible for an alarming increase in the incidence of human skin cancer, particularly among fair-skinned North Europeans.

Nutrition

Not only was life expectancy lower in the early 20th century but people were also shorter and lighter than they are today. Nutrition is the most significant factor affecting height and weight and the majority of people in the early 1900s had a poorer and plainer diet that, in some cases, was lacking in essential nutritional elements such as some vitamins and minerals. The average standard of nutrition has improved greatly in the last 50 years, although there is still deprivation and poverty. The health, development and growth of children is monitored from birth and continues throughout their school years so that those who may be at risk can be helped directly, for example by the provision of free school meals and vitamin/mineral supplements.

The consequences of greater affluence

The combination of a high-calorie diet and a lack of physical exercise has led to a huge rise in the incidence of obesity among Western peoples, the consequences of which pose a major health risk to those affected; a health risk that was almost unknown in the past. In Britain as in other Western countries, over-indulgence and affluence have become a threat to living a long and healthy life. However, it can be seen that overall, improvements in the environment and in living and working conditions, along with good nutrition and access to advanced medical care have resulted in a measurable increase in longevity over the past 100 years.

In fact, these improvements have probably had the greatest impact on the overall longevity of people in Britain. In some deprived inner city areas, where poverty, poor diet and bad housing are still prevalent, life expectancy is lower and people of all ages are more likely to succumb to illness and disease. Such areas of deprivation exist in most Western countries, echoing conditions that were formerly more widespread and show the significance to health and longevity of simple factors that can readily be changed.

In summary, people in 21st century Britain can expect to live longer and enjoy a better quality of life than their forebears of 100 years ago. Increased life expectancy has been achieved through improvements in the environment, nutrition and in health and medical care. However, environmental pollution, although of a different kind to that which prevailed a century ago, continues to threaten health and life expectancy, particularly through the incidence of cancer. It is known that many cancers have an environmental basis although the cause in any individual case often remains obscure. One in three people in modern Britain will contract a form of cancer at some stage in their lifetime, but the good news is that more people now are living for longer with the disease or surviving it completely, than in the past. This has been brought about by greatly improved surgical and medical treatments for the disease with new developments continually being made. Equally exciting is the research being carried out into the changes or mutations in cells that enable a cancer to grow. Scientists believe that they are close to understanding these key changes for several forms of cancer, holding out the hope that in the 21st century it will become possible to halt or reverse them and hence effect a cure.

Several diseases, including many cancers, are related to the process of ageing, i.e. they are more likely to affect people as they grow older. On the positive side is the fact that there are very many ways in which a person living today can reduce his or her chances of being affected. Not only is this the case but existing knowledge at this point in the 21st century also suggests that there are ways in which an individual can challenge the ageing process itself. Before considering these strategies, it is helpful to look at the possible causes of ageing. It has to be said that there are many scientific theories about this but those that are most widely accepted are described below.

Why Do We Age?

THERE is broad agreement about certain general aspects of the ageing process. The basic building blocks of the human body are the cells, different types of which form the various tissues and organs and perform the essential functions of life. These complex processes (called metabolism) are continually taking place within the cells of the human body. They both build up and break down products and create and utilise energy. Although essential for life, metabolism produces harmful by-products known as free radicals which are highly reactive and damaging to cells. In addition, external environmental pollution, both man-made (e.g. chemicals, tobacco smoke) and natural (e.g. radiation) further stimulates the production of free radicals within the body. Further harm can be caused by the faulty division of cells or by accidental damage, infection or disease.

The body employs a series of mechanisms to ensure the correct operation of all its numerous functions, to protect itself from harm and to repair any damage that may have occurred. These mechanisms, themselves part of metabolism and involving enzymes, hormones, genetic factors and the immune system, require energy in order to work. The energy molecules used by human cells are derived from food and normally require oxygen for their production. Energy and oxygen are the stuff of human life and everything else is dependent upon them. However, due to its involvement in the production of free radicals, oxygen is something of a double-edged sword, as will be seen from the discussion below.

In general, the mechanisms and processes of the human body, including those involved in protection and repair, operate at peak efficiency during youth and young adulthood. Changes and imbalances in the immune system, hormone and enzyme levels, production and utilisation of energy and in the operation of genetic material, occur after this time. It is these changes that are considered by scientists to be either directly or indirectly responsible for ageing and its effects. They are indirectly responsible when they cause a decline in the efficiency of the body's protective, defence and repair mechanisms, for example, enabling free radicals to have a more severe effect or disease to occur. They are directly responsible if they produce age-related effects. Hormone imbalances are probably the best example of this: for instance, the decline in oestrogen levels in menopausal and post-menopausal women is responsible for accelerating osteoporosis. It is helpful to examine some of the factors mentioned above a little more closely.

Free radicals and antioxidants

Free radicals are naturally occurring, unstable compounds that are very reactive. They have an additional proton or electron within their structure that allows them to freely attach to, and destroy, useful molecules and to damage cells. The majority of free radicals are produced within the body as a result of oxygen-driven metabolism. Among the most potent are toxic oxygen molecules that are able to oxidise useful agents within the body, including enzymes and other proteins and DNA, the genetic material of life itself. In fact, it has been suggested that each human cell is daily assaulted by several thousand free radical attacks. External or environmental substances that cause the production of free radicals include tobacco smoke, chemicals (paints, solvents, petroleum-based products, some cleaning fluids) exhaust emissions, alcohol, radiation, agricultural chemicals and fertilizers, and also sunlight.

Fortunately, the human body has defence mechanisms that can be employed to counter these attacks in the form of substances known as antioxidants. The body produces several known antioxidant enzymes, such as glutathione peroxidase and superoxide dismutase. Other substances, including some vitamins and minerals, are also active in this way. Environmental sources of free radicals should be avoided as far as possible by making sensible choices, especially with regard to those that lie directly within individual control, e.g. smoking and the drinking of alcohol.

Although it is impossible to prevent the production of free radicals within the body, it is possible to ensure that the diet contains plenty of natural antioxidant substances that are especially abundant in certain plant-based foods. Vitamins and minerals that have important antioxidant activity include vitamins C and E, selenium and sulphur. Two other groups of plant substances have also been found to be very important, carotenes and flavonoids. Various antioxidants are also available in supplement form.

In addition in being able to target free radicals directly, the body's defence and repair mechanisms are employed to put right any damage that occurs. One of the main theories of ageing proposes that, in time, the rate of free radical damage gradually overtakes the body's ability to counteract and repair it and so there is a general accumulation of adverse effects.

A branch of scientific research and development known as nanotechnology offers the hope that within the next 25 years it will become possible to use minute microprocessors to repair free radical damage directly. The theory is that tiny, cell-sized robots carrying living human material will be injected into a person's blood circulation, having first been programmed to proceed to a particular site and carry out repairs. The minute robots will theoretically be able to 'turn the clock back' and put right age-related damage that the person's own body can no longer cope with efficiently. Researchers in this field, working mainly in North America and Japan, certainly believe that this will become a reality. It is, however, likely to be an expensive technique and it remains to be seen whether it will become widely available to 'treat' natural ageing processes or whether it will be directed towards the treatment of serious diseases such as cancer.

The immune system

The immune system exists mainly to protect the body against invasion and infection by foreign particles such as bacteria and viruses. It also disposes of and controls obsolete and faulty host cells. It is composed of a number of different types of cells (leucocytes or white blood cells), chemicals and other molecules (special proteins called antibodies).

Chemistry of the immune system

The immune system has two main strands: natural or innate immunity that is present at birth and operates generally against almost any foreign substance; acquired or adaptive immunity that is generated as a result of an encounter with a specific foreign substance. There are three different types of leucocyte and all are involved in the operation of the immune system. Granulocytes comprise 70% of the total and they are involved in fighting bacterial and viral infections and possibly in allergy as well. Monocytes form the smallest component – 5% of the total number of leucocytes. They ingest and engulf bacteria, foreign bodies and dead body cells by a process known as phagocytosis. The third group, and probably the most important, are the lymphocytes which make up 25% of the total number.

There are two types of cells and both are vital in the operation of the immune system; B-cells or B-lymphocytes and T-cells or T-lymphocytes. B-cells produce *antibodies* that search out and bind with particular *antigens*. Antigen is the name given to any substance or particle that causes the formation of antibodies to neutralize its effect. Antigens are often protein substances that are regarded as 'foreign' and 'invading' by the immune system and so mobilize it into action. Good examples are bacteria and viruses. Antibodies are also protein substances that circulate in the blood. When an antibody finds its particular antigen, it fastens on to it somewhat in the manner of two pieces of a jigsaw puzzle fitting together. This neutralizes the antigen and renders it harmless. B-cells become activated when they come across particular antigens as in the event of invasion and infection by bacteria or viruses. They proliferate and secrete antibodies to counter the danger posed by the antigens. Following the event, some of the B-cells involved remain in the circulation, retaining a 'memory' of that particular antigen. Hence, should the antigen ever reinvade or be encountered again, mobilization of the antibody response will be even faster and greater than on the first occasion. This is acquired or adaptive immunity and is the principle behind vaccination.

T-cells circulate through the thymus gland where they differentiate. Like the B-cells, they are involved in the recognition of foreign antigens. In response to the presence of antigens, large numbers of T-cells are generated which secrete chemical compounds that assist in antibody production by the B-cells.

By combating disease-causing germs, getting rid of dead cells and aiding the recycling of useful molecules, the immune system preserves vitality and ensures the good health of the body.

Physiology of the immune system

The principal glands and tissues that are involved in the production and maintenance of the immune system are the bone marrow, lymph nodes, thymus gland and spleen. These all produce leucocytes and have additional functions as well. If they are not working effectively, it might be expected that this would contribute to a gradual deterioration in health. One of the principal theories behind ageing proposes that it occurs because of changes in the operation of the various elements of the immune system and a general decline in their level of effectiveness. There are several strands of evidence that support this theory and one of the most compelling is the observable alterations that occur in some of the glands and tissues that are involved.

Bone marrow

Bone marrow is the soft tissue that is found in the spaces of bones. In children (and other young mammals) all bone marrow, called red marrow, produces blood cells. In adults, the red marrow in long bones is gradually replaced by yellow marrow as ageing occurs. This is a fatty substance that does not produce blood cells. Hence in adults, red marrow is confined to the ribs, sternum, vertebrae and the ends of long bones such as the femur. The active part of red marrow is called myeloid tissue. This produces leucocytes and also erythroblasts, cells that develop into red blood corpuscles. All blood cells, including lymphocytes, differentiate from stem cells produced by the bone marrow. Some lymphocytes continue their development there, eventually maturing to become B-lymphocytes.

Lymph nodes

Lymph nodes are small, oval structures that occur at various points in the lymphatic system – a drainage network of vessels and valves that carries a clear, colourless fluid called lymph. Lymph is derived from the blood and consists mainly of water but, importantly, it carries lymphocytes and is eventually returned to the blood through the thoracic duct (one of two major vessels of the lymphatic system). Lymph nodes act as filters, by removing foreign particles. They also produce leucocytes and store lymphocytes. They are found grouped in several parts of the body including the neck, groin and armpit and can become swollen in the event of infection due to a proliferation of the cells involved in the immune response.

Thymus gland

The thymus gland is situated in the neck and forms a vital part of the body's defence system. It is especially important in childhood when it reaches the greatest extent of its development and size and is responsible for the production of lymphoid tissue and the laying down of the immune system. Some of the stem cells produced by the bone marrow migrate to the thymus gland where they undergo further differentiation and maturation to become T-lymphocytes. As has been seen, T-cells are vital for the effective operation of the immune system and they are dependent upon the thymus gland. The gland secretes thymosin, a peptide hormone which stimulates the maturation of the T-cells, along with a number of other chemical factors. At puberty, the thymus gradually begins to shrink in size and by adulthood it is very small indeed.

The spleen

The spleen is an egg-shaped, purple-coloured organ,

situated below the stomach which performs a number of different functions. It removes worn-out red blood cells, conserving their iron for further production in the bone marrow. It also stores red blood cells so that they can be released when needed. It is additionally involved in the production of leucocytes, including lymphocytes – the vital cells of the immune system as well as other blood components. Macrophages (one class of leucocytes) in the spleen are involved in the immune response by engulfing micro-organisms (bacteria and viruses) by phagocytosis. It is occasionally necessary to surgically remove the spleen, for example if it becomes ruptured due to accidental damage. In spite of the spleen's many functions, this can be performed without detriment although it is interesting to note that in the event, the lymph nodes increase in size. It is possible that the bone marrow also has to work harder if the spleen is removed.

It can be seen that there are significant changes in the bone marrow and thymus gland which are observable quite early on in a person's life. It is reasonable to suggest that these and other changes, such as a decline in the effectiveness and efficiency of the immune system, are at least partly responsible for ageing. Before leaving the immune system, one other piece of evidence for its involvement in ageing is provided by the occurrence of what are known as autoimmune diseases.

Auto immune diseases

These arise because, for some reason, the immune system loses its ability to distinguish between 'self' and 'non-self' and produces antibodies which attack the body's own tissues. A number of diseases are thought to be autoimmune disorders. In some of them, the precipitating factor seems to be initial infection – for example with streptococcal bacteria. The antibodies that the body produces to fight the bacteria can, in some cases, become 'confused' and attack body tissues. Hence these examples (of which the possible complications of rheumatic fever, i.e. heart valve damage may be one) can affect people of any age. However, other examples appear to be more common in older people and it can be inferred that they may arise because an ageing immune system is no longer working so efficiently. Possible examples include rheumatoid arthritis, maturity-onset diabetes, lupus erythematosus and systemic lupus erythematosus, and Grave's disease. Autoimmune diseases may be an extreme example of what can happen when the immune system goes awry. It is certainly possible that age-related effects occur partly because of slighter and less dramatic changes in the operation of the system.

Hormonal factors

The hormonal or endocrine system is highly complex. It involves a number of different glands and organs that produce chemical substances that control body functions and interact with one another to a greater or lesser extent. One of the most widely-held theories about ageing proposes that it occurs because of hormonal imbalances that arise over time in parts of the system. The glands and hormones that are believed by some researchers to be most involved are the pituitary (growth hormone and hormones that stimulate the sex organs to produce their hormones); thyroid (thyroxine and triiodothyronine – essential for the regulation of metabolism and growth); thymus (thymos in which stimulates the maturation of T-lymphocytes); pineal (melatonin – involved in the regulation of internal 'body clocks' and circadian rhythms). Also important are oestrogen, produced by the ovaries and possibly testosterone, the male sex hormone released by cells in the testicles. A close examination of these glands and hormones reveals just how complex and far-reaching are their activities. It is highly probable that they are, indeed, involved in the processes of ageing and probably in ways which are, as yet, not fully understood.

Pituitary gland (and hypothalamus)

The pituitary gland or hypophysis is a small but very important gland situated at the base of the brain, beneath an area called the hypothalamus. It is arguably the lynchpin of the endocrine system, for it has two lobes which each secrete hormones that act on other glands and control many different functions. The pituitary produces growth hormone or somatotrophin which, by means of protein synthesis, controls the growth of long bones in children and enlargement and repair of muscles and bones in adult life. The pitutary also produces gonadotrophins which are hormones that act on the sex organs and stimulate them to produce their hormones. Thyroid-stimulating hormones released by the pituitary act upon the thyroid gland, prompting it to produce and release its own hormones. The pituitary gland is itself regulated by releasing factors and hormones that are secreted by the hypothalamus, an area of the brain. Some experts believe that the pituitary gland declines in efficiency with time and that this has far-reaching consequences for the body's hormonal systems and is responsible for ageing. The cause of pituitary gland inefficiency is thought to be a gradual and progressive disturbance in the body's internal 'clocks' (*see* pineal gland and melatonin, page 30).

Thyroid gland

The thyroid gland is situated at the base and front of the neck and secretes two iodine-rich hormones, thyroxine and triiodothyronine. These are essential for the regulation of metabolism and growth. Overactivity of the thyroid gland, or hyperthyroidism, results in a high metabolic rate with increased utilisation of oxygen and occurs in Graves disease (*see* autoimmune diseases, page 27). Due to its complex effects upon metabolism, some researchers believe that changes in the operation of the thyroid gland and its hormones are partly responsible for ageing.

Thymus gland

The importance of the thymus gland to the establishment of the immune system has already been described (*see* page 21). The gland produces the hormone thymosin which stimulates the maturation of the T-lymphocytes which are vital for the effectiveness of the immune system. The thymus gland begins to shrink at puberty and the concentration of thymosin declines. Those who hold to the theory that a declining immune system is the key to ageing believe that the decline in thymosin plays a significant part in the process.

Pineal gland

The pineal gland is a somewhat mysterious, small tissue mass located almost centrally within the brain, which secretes the hormone melatonin. Melatonin is secreted mainly during the hours of darkness (the pineal gland itself contains light-sensitive cells and has nerve connections with the eyes) and so greater amounts of the hormone are released during the winter months. It is connected with the operation of biological clocks and, in many vertebrate animals, is involved in seasonal activities, especially breeding. For example, it has a role in changes in skin pigmentation and hence the breeding colours assumed by many animals.

Melatonin is apparently involved in a way that is not understood in the operation of circadian rhythms, which are the regular changes that occur in an animal's behaviour and physiology in each 24-hour period. Hence it is somehow involved in cycles and rhythms linked to the passage of time. In people, the secretion of melatonin apparently declines with age. Some researchers believe that ageing itself occurs because the operation of internal body clocks goes awry and that the decline in melatonin is a significant factor in this process. (*See* hormonal anti-ageing treatments, page 147).

Sex hormones

The male sex hormones are called androgens. These are produced by the testicles, of which the principal and best known one is testosterone. Androgens are also produced in small amounts by the adrenal glands (a pair of important hormone-secreting glands located above each kidney) and by the female ovaries. Androgens are responsible for the development of the male sex organs and for the appearance of the secondary sexual characteristics at puberty. They are also necessary for the production of sperm, a process which continues throughout life, from puberty into old age. Androgens are responsible for the sex drive (libido) in males and play a part in behavioural characteristics such as aggressiveness and competitiveness.

Testosterone is produced throughout life at a more or less constant level. However, there is a very slight reduction in the level in older age. Also, the amount produced by different individuals varies quite considerably so it is not possible to ascertain a correct or normal level. Some researchers believe that testosterone does not work as effectively in middle-aged men, even though the level at which it is produced has not significantly altered, and that this is responsible for a number of ageing effects. Testosterone supplementation is sometimes given to counteract these effects (*see* hormonal treatments, page 147) but it is a controversial therapy.

The female sex hormones are the oestrogens and progestogens, mainly secreted by the ovaries. Oestrogen is also manufactured in small amounts by the adrenal glands and female fatty tissue. A very small quantity is produced by the testicles in men. Oestrogen is responsible for the maturation of the female sex organs and for the development of the secondary sexual characteristics at puberty. Interaction between oestrogen and progesterone and pituitary hormones is responsible for the implementation of the female reproductive cycles in the ovaries (ovarian cycle) and womb (menstrual cycle). A lack of these hormones, particularly oestrogen, during and after the menopause, is responsible for the best understood age-related effects and symptoms seen in women. Hormone replacement therapy is routinely given to women to alleviate menopausal symptoms but it also helps to reverse some ageing effects as well.

Genetic factors

It is commonly accepted that genetic factors play a complex part in ageing and longevity, although their precise role is open to dispute. Longevity does run in some families in whom it must certainly be genetically determined. To a certain extent, everyone can gain some idea of their potential life span by considering that of their parents and grandparents – a fact which is taken into account by insurance companies. In some simple animals such as fruit flies, scientists believe they have discovered the existence of an 'ageing gene' which, when manipulated, extends the normal life span of the flies by as much as 50%. There has been speculation as to whether such genes might exist in human beings and other higher mammals.

In August 2001, scientists announced that they had discovered a group of so-called 'Methuselah' genes which, they believed, held the key to long life. They had studied 137 people aged 100 years or over and had discovered that all these people shared a common section of genes, located on chromosome 4. Scientists believe that these genes, if 'switched on', are able to combat age-related diseases and enable their owners to enjoy an extended and, more importantly, healthy, lifespan. It is thought that about ten genes are involved but it is not known exactly which ones they are out of a possible 100 to 500 on the strand of chromosomes. Work is now underway to isolate the key group of genes involved. Interestingly, the centenarians studied did not necessarily have particularly healthy lifestyles and came from a wide variety of cultures and social backgrounds. It seems that most of us do not, at present, have activated Methuselah genes as relatively few people live to be a healthy 100 years old.

However, scientists believe that gene manipulation may open up this possibility to more people in the future. Methuselah genes have already been discovered in simple nematode worms and in fruit flies. In 1999, scientists announced that, using genetic manipulation, they had 'created' a strain of mice that lived longer than genetically unaltered mice by up to one-third of the normal lifespan. Mice are, of course, warm-blooded mammals like ourselves. Scientists working on the human Methuselah gene project have stressed that their aim is to promote healthy old age rather than longevity itself. But it may be the case that the 21st century comes to be seen as the best time in history for humans to be growing old!

Genes are carried on *chromosomes*, rod-like structures contained within the nucleus of cells. Each chromosome consists mainly of a large molecule of DNA (deoxyribonucleic acid) which comprises two twisted chains, connected together by ladder-like rungs in a double helix. The chains consist of sugar-phosphate molecules while the rungs are pairs of nitrogenous bases which join together in a particular way. When DNA divides (as in cell division) the chains first unravel and then each serves as a template for the synthesis and copying of a new strand, ending up with two daughter molecules. One of these is retained within each half of the nucleus as the cell divides. At the end of each DNA molecule (and hence each chromosome) are specialized strands of DNA. These are called *telomeres* and they consist of a more simple, repeating sequence than that found in the bulk of the molecule. Their purpose is to ensure that the DNA is accurately copied each time the cell divides and, in most human cells, they become progressively shorter with every division. Eventually, the telomeres become so short that accurate division can no longer take place and the cell dies.

The activity of the telomeres is governed by a group of enzymes (proteins) called reverse transcriptases or telomerases. These manufacture the telomeres and stick them onto the ends of the chromosomal DNA. The gene for telomerase is present in all human cells but it appears that the activity of the protein usually declines, causing the cells to age and eventually die. The exceptions are the so-called immortal cells – reproductive cells and cancer cells – in which the telomeres remain long and the level of telomerase is high. These cells continue to divide and do not die and this is the reason why cancer cells are so dangerous and destructive. In recent years, scientists have isolated a human gene for an enzyme called telomerase reverse transcriptase or hTRT which is found only in immortal cells. It has been discovered that if this gene is introduced into cultures of ordinary human cells, they start to make telomerase. The dormant telomerase gene in these cells appears to be activated with the result that the telomeres are lengthened. These ordinary cells then continue to divide instead of ageing and dying as would be the normal course of events. Some researchers believe that this discovery will eventually be used to halt the normal processes of ageing, at cellular level. However, other research suggests that doing this might actually increase the risks of cancer while some experts remain unconvinced of the significance of telomerase in ageing.

A more promising future development may be the manipulation and reduction of telomerase to halt the progression of cancer. Considerable research effort is being devoted to this and it is hoped that it will eventually provide a useful treatment for this disease.

Production and utilisation of energy
This is a somewhat vague and all-embracing heading which, once again, includes all the complex

metabolic processes that are necessary for life. The efficiency of these processes declines with the passage of time, allowing age-related effects to occur. Energy use and production ultimately depend upon fuel (derived from food and digestion) and oxygen (from respiration).

Digestive problems tend to become more common in middle and older age and absorption of the simple, breakdown products of digestion is often compromised. Respiration describes the whole process by which air is drawn into and out of the lungs, during which oxygen is absorbed into the bloodstream and carbon dioxide and water are given off. External respiration is the actual process of breathing and the exchange of gases (oxygen in, carbon dioxide out) that takes place in the lungs. Internal respiration is the process by which oxygen is given up from the blood circulation to the tissues in all parts of the body, while carbon dioxide is taken up, transported back to the lungs and eliminated. The process of drawing air into the lungs is known as inhalation or inspiration and expelling it out is exhalation or expiration – all more commonly called breathing. All aspects of respiration can become less effective with time, from the mechanical processes of breathing to the exchange of gases between tissues and the bloodstream.

Production of energy actually occurs within cells themselves and involves a complex series of biochemical reactions which are controlled by special proteins called enzymes and which require oxygen. The biochemical reactions are of a cyclical nature and use glucose molecules or fatty acids (the final products of the digestion of carbohydrates and fats) as fuel. These undergo a series of changes that result in the production of molecules of energy called ATP that the cells can use directly. Molecules of carbon dioxide are given off as waste products to be passed out of the cell. These biochemical reactions are essential to provide the energy for all life processes to occur. Some researchers believe that problems with energy hold the key to the ageing process.

Although the main factors believed to be at work in ageing have been described above under separate headings for the sake of convenience, it can be appreciated that they are all closely connected with each other. The processes of life are interdependent and it is likely that ageing itself occurs because of some or all of the aspects covered above. If there are many causes there may also be many solutions and, as yet, no one has the key to immortality. There are, however, several anti-ageing strategies that can be employed and which increase the chances of living a long, healthy and active life. Before turning to these, it is useful to examine the commonly-held perceptions about ageing and to expose the truth (or otherwise) of what it is that so many people fear.

Facts and Myths
about Older Age

I N A recent television programme, a group of young people were brought together with some who were elderly to explore the misconceptions about old age and the issues of ageism. Most of the young people were in their 20s and almost all of them believed that worthwhile life was over by about the age of 50! They thought that older people were unattractive, beset with infirmities and medical conditions, no longer had fun or knew how to enjoy themselves and were past their best in their working life and should move aside to make room for the young. They also believed that sex could not be enjoyed by older people in the same way as it was by those who were young.

These young people were confronted by a group of mature and elderly citizens who were living proof that their misconceptions were wrong on every count. The older group were, in fact, taking part in many more activities, including vigorous sports, than the younger ones. They had energy, expertise and experience which they were using in very many different ways, along with the self-confidence to face up to new challenges in life. As for having no enjoyment of sex, most asserted that this area of life was better than it had ever been when they were young! All of them believed that the key to a successful and enjoyable older age lay within themselves and that it was achievable with a little effort and determination – qualities which they felt were lacking in the younger generation!

Surveys show that the type of misconceptions outlined above are commonplace, especially among young people. Naturally, some readjustment in thinking inevitably takes place as each individual progresses from youth to older age. However, other ideas are more entrenched and it is common to hear some condition or other being dismissed as 'just old age', the inference being that there is nothing that can be done and the person will just have to put up with it. Obviously, physical changes *do* occur and there *are* illnesses and conditions that are more common in older age. However, illness can strike at any time in life and the good news is that a great deal can be done to prevent natural bodily changes from causing problems in later life. An overview of some of the more common of these is given below.

Skeleton, joints and muscles

Up to the age of about 30, calcium is stored in the bones and there should normally be plenty available for the replacement of worn out bone cells in order to ensure that the bones remain strong. It is essential for growing children and young people to eat a diet that is rich in calcium as this is the stage when the quality and strength of the skeleton is being determined. After the age of 30, there is a gradual decline in the amount of calcium resulting in a steady thinning of the bones. This process is accelerated in women at the time of the menopause and is connected with a sharp decline in the level of the hormone, oestrogen.

When thinning of the bones is especially severe, the bones become brittle and subject to fractures and this condition is known as osteoporosis. Osteoporosis affects more women than men due to the effects of the menopause and because the female skeleton is smaller and lighter in the first place.

The joints are subjected to a great deal of use throughout life, much which is unavoidable and can be termed general 'wear and tear'. With the passage of time, the joints can become progressively stiffer and movements are less free and more restricted than in youth. This is due to the fact that there are gradual changes in the quantity of lubricating fluid and tissue (including cartilage and ligaments) with age. Wear and tear may cause the bone surfaces to become roughened, with a loss of the covering of cartilage and lubricating synovial fluid, leading to the development of arthritis. There are very many different forms of arthritis but one of the most common types, arising in middle and older age, is osteoarthritis. Arthritic changes are extremely common and there appear to be many contributory factors implicated in their occurrence. Although the degenerative changes cannot be reversed, there are very many ways in which the condition of the joints can be safeguarded, and therapies are available to treat arthritis symptoms.

There is a gradual loss of muscle mass and strength with age but the extent of this can be offset by remaining active and taking regular exercise. A fit, elderly person can have muscles that are in a much better condition than those of a younger person who does not bother to exercise. There is a tendency for muscle to be replaced by fatty tissue and in women, the amount increases considerably over that which is present in youth. Once again, regular exercise and an active lifestyle can help to slow this process down and encourage good health in older age.

The heart and circulation

Heart and circulatory disease is one of the most significant causes of premature death in Britain, and while it used to affect mainly older people, it is now striking at those in younger age groups. It is well known that there is a strong link between the western lifestyle, particularly with regard to diet, and heart and circulatory disease. Some slight degeneration in the circulatory system may be an inevitable consequence of ageing but the situation is greatly aggravated by consuming a diet high in saturated fat which causes 'furring' of the arteries (atherosclerosis).

This type of disease is uncommon among the peoples of the Far East who eat a diet that is protective of the heart and circulation. The heart is basically a muscular pump containing a built-in pacemaker which directs it to keep on beating throughout life. The operation of the pump may become less efficient with age and the best way of preventing this and protecting the heart is through regular exercise.

Other organs – lungs, liver, kidneys

The lungs are a pair of fibrous, elastic sacs which have folded surfaces internally to provide a large surface area for the exchange of gases. Air enters the body through the windpipe or trachea which branches into two bronchi (bronchus), one to each lung. Further branching then occurs into finer tubes called bronchioles. The bronchioles divide further into alveoli. It is known that people quickly lose the efficient method of breathing, using the diaphragm, that is natural during childhood and instead resort to chest breathing which is less effective and fails to empty the lungs properly. The result of this is that part of the capacity of the lungs is not used and eventually, with ageing, they lose some of their natural elasticity. Once this occurs, the lungs are no longer capable of expanding to the extent that they did in youth and so the amount of air taken in (and hence, available oxygen) is reduced. It is well worth relearning the art of correct breathing during adult life to maintain the natural elasticity of the lungs. (*See* section on Exercise, page 105).

The liver is both a very important organ, and a gland, performing many functions which are critical in regulating metabolic processes. It is a large, four-lobed organ, situated in the top right-hand part of the abdominal cavity. Two major blood vessels supply the liver. The hepatic artery delivers oxygenated blood while the hepatic portal vein carries digested food absorbed into the blood from the stomach directly to the liver. Among its many functions, the liver converts excess glucose (the end product of carbohydrate digestion) to glycogen (a more complex molecule, also called animal starch) for storage as a food reserve.

Excess amounts of amino acids (the end products of protein digestion) are converted to the waste compound urea, containing nitrogen, which is then transported in the blood to the kidneys where it is eliminated. Bile is produced in the liver and stored in the gall bladder from where it is released and used in fat digestion and the absorption of nutrients. Lipolysis, which is the breakdown of lipids (fats, oils, waxes) from fat digestion into fatty acids, (essential molecules that are used by the body in a number of ways) takes place in the liver. Several poisons (toxins) are broken down (detoxified) by the liver, a good example being alcohol. Since the hepatic portal vein carries ingested products directly from the gut, the liver is the first important port of call for all material that is taken in by mouth, whether helpful or harmful.

The liver manufactures blood clotting substances and processes worn-out red blood cells, removing the haemoglobin and storing it as iron for future use. Vitamin A is manufactured and stored and the liver also stores vitamins B_{12}, D, E and K. The chemical and biochemical activity of the liver is so great that significant energy is generated and this organ is a major contributor of heat to the body. In older age, the liver may become less efficient in performing its functions such as that of detoxification. This means that care has to be taken with alcohol consumption and with over-the-counter and prescription drugs as the liver is more vulnerable to damage.

The kidneys are a pair of organs and glands that are positioned in the back of the abdomen below the diaphragm. Their function is to remove nitrogen-containing wastes (mainly urea) from the blood and adjust the concentrations of various salts. They act as filters of the blood and produce urine which is eliminated to the outside via the bladder. The kidneys contain numerous fine, folded tubules (called nephrons) and they receive about 1,000–2,000 litres of blood each day and process 150–200 litres of filtrate. This results in the daily production of about 1.5 litres of urine. The kidneys may work less efficiently in older age resulting in a slower removal of toxins from the blood. The urinary system may be more prone to infection in older age. Some nutritional elements and dietary supplements can help to boost kidney and liver function.

Digestive system

In general, digestion and the absorption of food from the gut becomes less effective in older age and people may experience minor problems, such as indigestion, a little more frequently. Sometimes, people find that a food that they were readily able to eat in the past begins to cause upset and unfortunately, this may mean having to avoid something that would otherwise be enjoyed. Older people are vulnerable to deficiencies in various nutritional elements due to malabsorption and one way of overcoming this is by the use of supplements. In old age, metabolic rate slows and fewer calories are required than in youth. However, as at any age, this greatly depends upon the amount of energy being expended so that a fit, active, elderly person will need more food than someone of the same age with a more sedentary lifestyle.

The senses – hearing, sight, taste and smell

It is well known that the sense of hearing begins to deteriorate in older age. Some people merely experience a slight loss of hearing which is not a problem but in others, the deafness is more profound. Treatment depends upon cause but as long as there is no nerve damage it is usually possible to improve the situation, often by fitting a hearing aid. However, it is quite common for a build-up of hardened ear wax to be the cause of temporary deafness in an older person, in which case the problem is solved by syringing the ears.

The eyes are subject to various physical changes during ageing which affect vision. These changes often affect the lens (the structure which focuses light rays) or the muscles that control it. There is a natural tendency towards long-sightedness during ageing (in which light is focused behind, instead of on, the retina where the image should normally be formed).

This is simply treated by the wearing of glasses with convex lenses for reading and other close work. Age-related problems affecting the muscles that control the lens are nowadays often successfully treated by means of corrective micro-surgery. Cataract formation is a common problem in elderly people but is fortunately one which is highly amenable to treatment. It is caused by natural changes in the crystalline protein components of the lens which cause this structure to become visibly opaque, leading to loss of vision. It is treated by surgical removal of the cataract which is highly successful in restoring sight.

The sense of taste is conferred by taste buds which are minute sensory receptors located on the tongue and in the back of the mouth. They are stimulated by the presence of dissolved food in the saliva and messages are sent via nerves to the brain where the information is interpreted and perceived. Sweetness, sourness and saltiness are among the tastes that can be perceived and these become dulled as ageing progresses, although the extent to which this occurs is probably variable.

However, the decline in the perception of saltiness is something which an elderly person should take into account as it is all too easy to add excess salt to food without realizing that one is doing so.

The sense of smell, or olfaction, is closely related to that of taste. The nasal cavities of the nose are lined with moist mucous membranes in which the minute olfactory sensory receptors are located. These are stimulated by chemicals contained in inhaled air which dissolve in the moisture of the mucous membrane lining.

Each olfactory receptor is connected to the brain via the olfactory nerve and it is here that the smell is interpreted and identified. There may be some slight deadening of the sense of smell in older age but, as it happens gradually, it is not usually noticeable.

The brain – intellect and memory

The brain is subject to age-related changes in a number of different ways. From a relatively early stage in adult life there is a net loss of brain cells which are not regenerated or replaced. Most people probably do not notice these changes, which are slight and gradual. However, in middle and older age, many people experience some degree of forgetfulness which is a reflection of ageing processes affecting the brain. Some degree of short-term memory loss is very common in more advanced old age but the extent to which people are affected is variable. Decision-making and problem-solving, along with the understanding and assimilation of complex information, may take longer at an advanced age but once again, the extent to which individuals are affected varies from one person to another. Many old people are extremely 'sharp' and are scarcely affected by these changes. Intelligence does not alter with age and neither does the ability to learn new skills, although the time required may be greater than was the case in youth.

An alarmingly high number of elderly people suffer from some form of dementia, either senile dementia or Alzheimer's disease. Senile dementia is an organic mental disorder characterized by general atrophy of the brain. There is a gradual deterioration with loss of short-term memory, impaired judgement, confusion, emotional outbursts and irritability. The severity of the condition is variable. Alzheimer's disease is the commonest form of dementia and can affect people in younger age groups, as well as the elderly. Degenerative changes take place in the cerebral cortex of the brain with the formation of plaques of tissue. There is progressive loss of memory, disintegration of personality and eventual inability to perform basic functions. Dementia is discussed in greater detail in a later section of this book. (*See* age-related conditions, page 184). There are many ways in which intellectual faculties can be safeguarded in order to combat the natural effects of ageing. (*See* brain exercises, page 122).

Sexual capabilities

Men retain their reproductive capability throughout life and the level of the sex hormone, testosterone, falls only slightly with increasing age. There may be some slight loss of libido and a man may find it harder to reach and maintain an erection with advancing age. However, problems of sexual performance are often related to some other cause (e.g. a condition for which drugs are being taken or stress) rather than to ageing as such. The loss of oestrogen at the menopause affects vaginal secretions in women and lack of lubrication can be a physical problem preventing sexual enjoyment, although one which is readily overcome. Women may also experience a loss of libido after the menopause but this is by no means always the case. Hormone replacement therapy or other supplements often prove helpful in overcoming problems of sexual performance.

Men and women who have enjoyed an active sex life usually continue to be sexually active in older age. Surveys have not revealed an average age at which people cease to be interested in sex and this area of life is governed by individual preference at every stage.

Lay the foundations for a long and healthy life. Whatever age you are, now is the time to start!

There is, as yet, no magic formula or elixir of youth that can extend life. There are, however, a number of biological compounds and supplements which may slow down the processes of ageing and some of these stand up to scientific scrutiny better than others. Anti-ageing supplements are discussed in a later section of this book but it should be realized that the use of these products is often controversial and they are usually expensive. The medical profession is, on the whole, a conservative one. Anti-ageing products are not usually available on the NHS, unless they are of proven benefit in treating an age-related disease. Some formulations may be available privately, often at considerable cost. Others, which fall into the category of health or herbal supplements such as Ginkgo biloba, are widely available and more reasonably priced.

The good news is that, for most people, preparing for a long and healthy life does not depend upon the size of their bank balance but upon choices that lie within individual control. Sadly, the exceptions to this are those people who, in 21st century Britain, are still living in extreme poverty. Research has shown that these people have a lower than average life expectancy. Children born into poverty are more likely to contract infections and conditions which may be life-threatening. Many poor people in Britain feel that they lack the financial means to safeguard their health and longevity and it is likely that government initiatives will continue to be necessary to improve their situation.

So what steps can an ordinary person take to increase his or her chances of leading a longer and healthy life? The most important measures involve adopting a way of living which is mind and body conscious, i.e. aimed at promoting good health, preventing ill-health and, as far as possible, combating age-related conditions. The most significant areas of life to examine are diet and such lifestyle factors as taking exercise and reducing risks and stress. Sensible use of supplements, depending upon your age and sex, will enhance your anti-ageing regime.

It is a good idea to adopt anti-ageing strategies in youth but, of course, human nature being the way it is, very few people do this! Starting young is obviously going to confer some advantage but it is important to realize that you can make a difference at every age. Evidently, if someone is just starting an anti-ageing plan in his or her eighties, the difference is likely to be in the quality of life rather than its quantity or extent – but it is still well worth making the change. The message is that whatever age we may be, it is never too late to incorporate anti-ageing strategies into our lifestyle.

In the following sections, we shall look at the ways and means by which this can be achieved.

Anti-ageing Nutrition

A POPULAR saying states that 'You are what you eat' and evidence is now overwhelming that we influence our health and longevity through the food that we consume on a day-to-day basis. By choosing our food wisely, we can promote anti-ageing in two ways. Firstly, by reducing our chances of contracting certain diseases and conditions that threaten the extent and quality of life and secondly, by directly supporting the body's anti-ageing mechanisms through eating foods that are known to be beneficial.

The first way basically means accepting and practising what has come to be known as healthy eating. In order to understand this concept, it is necessary to examine the different elements in food and the body's requirements for them. We can then see why the western diet is considered to be both unhealthy and detrimental to a person's chances of leading a long and healthy life.

The human body requires food to provide energy for all life processes and for growth, repair and maintenance of cells and tissues, including those of the immune system, vital for warding off disease and the effects of ageing. Food consists of, or contains, three main groups of substances which are needed by the body in differing amounts: carbohydrates, proteins and fats. In addition, the body requires fibre (derived from plants) which is essential in promoting good health and in preventing a number of life-threatening diseases. Vitamins and minerals are needed on a daily basis in small amounts and, as will be seen later, some of them are vital in the fight against ageing. While it is best to fulfil vitamin and mineral needs from the diet, supplements are helpful for certain groups of people.

Carbohydrates

Carbohydrates consist of either simple or more complex forms of sugar molecules of which the most basic is glucose. All carbohydrates are eventually broken down by digestive processes into glucose which is absorbed into the bloodstream and utilised by the body in various ways. The more simple the carbohydrate or sugar molecule in the food, the more rapid is the process of digestion and absorption of glucose into the bloodstream. It may be used immediately, particularly if energy demands are high as during vigorous exercise. Athletes often take pure glucose for this purpose.

Starches are complex carbohydrates built up of chains of glucose molecules. They take longer to be broken down by digestive processes and hence provide a more gradual, sustained supply of glucose. The body generally contains sufficient reserves of glucose to meet the total energy requirements for one day's activity. If there is a lack of glucose, the body is able to manufacture it in the liver using glycerol (from fats) and amino acids (from proteins) as raw materials. Conversely, as previously noted, excess glucose is converted by the liver into the complex carbohydrate glycogen, or animal starch. This is stored in liver and muscle cells and used when there is a lack of available glucose in the blood.

Processed foodstuffs such as sweets, biscuits, cakes, chocolates and sauces usually consist mainly of simple sugars that merely provide the body with calories, i.e. energy molecules in the form of glucose. Unfortunately, people in the UK and in western countries enjoy these highly palatable foods and eat them to excess and to the exclusion of more helpful foods. Excess consumption contributes towards life-shortening conditions such as obesity, diabetes mellitus and atherosclerosis, and is a major cause of tooth decay.

On the other hand, foods such as cereals, grains, bread, pasta, potatoes, vegetables and fruits are largely composed of starch and also contain helpful fibre, vitamins and minerals. Nutritional experts recommend that complex carbohydrates in the form of starchy foods should make up 60%–70% of overall daily intake. These should be in the form of wholemeal bread, cereals, whole grains, wholegrain rice, brown pasta and potatoes (especially with their skins) which all have a high fibre content. These are more satisfying and filling than the white varieties of the same foods and reduce any tendency to overeat. They can thus help to combat obesity and maintain a healthy weight.

Proteins

Proteins are the structural components of the body forming the basis of cells, tissues and organs. The units of which they are composed are called amino acids and these are usually arranged in lines to make up molecules known as polypeptides. Proteins are broken down by digestion into amino acids, the form in which they are absorbed. There are 20 basic amino acids that can be arranged in a huge number of different ways. Most proteins consist of more than one polypeptide chain and there are vast numbers in the body, each with a unique structure but all made from the 'pool' of 20 amino acids. In addition to being structural molecules, proteins are used in the body for storage, as messengers (e.g. hormones), as carriers (e.g. the globin in the haemoglobin of red blood cells which transport oxygen) and as facilitators or catalysts of biochemical, metabolic reactions (e.g. enzymes).

The body is able to manufacture 12 of the 20 amino acids but the remainder, called the 'essential amino acids' must be obtained from food. Proteins are widely found in foods of both plant and animal origin. Plant sources include beans, peas, pulses, whole grains, nuts and seeds. Red meat, poultry, fish, milk, cheese, yoghurt and eggs are the main animal sources. Red meat is traditionally regarded as first-class protein and is a good source of essential amino acids and iron. But nutritionists recommend limiting the consumption of red meat to once or perhaps twice a week and choosing foods that are high in protein but low in saturated fat (e.g. pulses, beans, nuts and seeds, low fat dairy produce, poultry breast meat) instead. Protein should form 10%–15% of the total daily calorie intake and so only a small amount is needed at each meal. Oily fish such as mackerel, herring, sardines, salmon, trout, pilchards and tuna are both excellent sources of protein and also the helpful form of fat (see below). These should be eaten at least two or three times a week as the oils that they contain protect against heart disease and some other conditions. Peas and beans are not only good sources of vegetable protein but help to reduce levels of blood cholesterol.

Fats

Fats in the form of organic compounds called lipids are widely found in plant and animal cells and perform many vital functions. They are an important, high energy store, having twice the calorific value of carbohydrates, and provide insulation and cushioning. Fats contain fatty acid molecules and may be either saturated or unsaturated, depending upon their chemical structure. Saturated fats are solid while unsaturated ones have a softer or more liquid consistency.

Fatty acids perform three major functions in the human body. They are vital components of the membrane that surrounds all types of tissue cell and controls the passage of substances both into and out of the cell. Compounds derived from fatty acids serve as hormones and chemical messengers within and between cells, tissues and organs. Fatty acids are stored (joined to other molecules) inside cells as fuel reserves that can be broken down when required to release large quantities of energy.

The best known example of a saturated fat is cholesterol which is manufactured by the liver from saturated fatty acids. Cholesterol is an essential substance, being a component of cell membranes and involved in the production of steroid hormones and bile salts. However, the body is capable of supplying the necessary amount of cholesterol from a very small dietary intake. In western countries, the diet is high in saturated fats which are found in red meat, full fat dairy products and eggs but, more importantly, are widely used in the manufacture of processed foods. In addition, consumption of helpful fibre-rich foods that may bind to cholesterol, tends to be low. The result is that too much cholesterol ends up circulating in the blood and if this situation is prolonged, there is a high risk of furring and partial blocking of the arteries – atherosclerosis or atheroma. These conditions are a causal factor in heart disease and heart attack, angina and stroke which are a major, age-related cause of disability and premature death. Scientific studies have revealed that an alarmingly high number of young school children in the UK show evidence of early atherosclerosis. There is great concern that without a change in diet, those affected will be at high risk of heart and circulatory disease in young adult life.

We have seen that fats are essential for human health but in order to prevent disease and indeed, to promote good health and longevity, they need to be in the right form. Unsaturated fats are of two types; polyunsaturated and monounsaturated. The polyun-saturated forms include a group which is termed the 'essential fatty acids' because human beings can only obtain them from food. Good sources of polyunsatu-rated fats are oily fish (mackerel, salmon, trout, tuna, herring, sardines, anchovies), various vegetable oils (safflower, sunflower, flaxseed oil, corn, grapeseed, soya bean, perilla oil and linseed oil), and also flax seeds (sesame seeds, sunflower seeds, walnuts, among others). Oily fish is protective against heart disease and studies have shown that people whose diet is rich in these fish, such as the Japanese and Inuit (Eskimos), have a very low incidence. Some of these oils (fish oil, flaxseed oil, linseed oil, perilla oil) have anti-inflammatory, anti-allergic properties. Sufferers from eczema, psoriasis, rheumatoid arthritis and osteoarthritis may be helped by increasing their intake of beneficial oils. The oils may also reduce the risk of contracting certain forms of cancer (ovarian and bowel).

The overall consumption of helpful forms of fat should be in the order of 25% of daily intake of calories and should not exceed 30%. A very low fat or no-fat diet is as unhealthy and damaging as eating too much fat. As we have seen, most adults in western countries eat an excess of fat, much of it 'hidden' in processed foods. A good way of reducing the amount is to switch to semi-skimmed or skimmed milk and low fat dairy produce, choose low fat cooking methods and avoid highly processed, 'convenience' foods as much as possible. It must also be appreciated that diet alone cannot protect an individual against heart disease but it can significantly reduce risk. It is well known that lifestyle factors such as lack of exercise and smoking are the other significant parts of the risk equation, but these are factors that also lie within individual control and are very much a part of anti-ageing.

Fibre
Fibre is found in the cell walls of plants and so is present in greater or lesser amounts in all plant-based

foods, other than those that have been highly refined by processing. Lack of dietary fibre in the UK and other western countries has been identified as a significant cause of ill health, being linked with a number of serious illnesses and conditions. Some of these are directly linked to the digestive tract while others affect other body systems and organs. Hence a lack of dietary fibre can have far-reaching consequences.

Diseases include:

1 Digestive – bowel cancer (cancer of the large intestine, colon and rectum), constipation, diverticulosis.
2 Heart and circulatory, linked with high consumption of saturated fats – atherosclerosis and atheroma; varicose veins.
3 Others – one of the dietary factors contributing towards the development of obesity, kidney stones (some forms), gallstones and diabetes mellitus.

These conditions are rare in people who eat a fibre-rich, wholefood diet that is largely plant-based. Fibre, also known as roughage, occurs in various forms depending upon the nature of the source plant. One of the most ubiquitous forms is cellulose which is the main constituent of the cell walls of plants. The most readily available sources are foods containing wholewheat bran such as wholemeal flour and bread, wholemeal pasta and also brown rice (which retains the husk). Cellulose is insoluble fibre, i.e. it does not break down in water. It is able to bind to water and adds bulk to the waste products of digestion, promoting the efficient operation of the bowel. Other forms of fibre such as pectins (found in fruits, citrus peel, vegetables) and hemicelluloses (found in oat bran, seeds, peas, beans, grains, vegetables and fruits) are water soluble. They have gel-producing effects, are able to bind to cholesterol and excess bile salts and promote a slower release of food from the stomach, allowing more time for nutrients to be broken down and absorbed. Hemicelluloses are important sources of helpful fatty acids, provide energy for cells in the lining of the colon and are believed to have anti-cancer activity. Porridge (from oats) is a well-known form of hemicellulose. Eating a bowl of porridge at breakfast time has been shown not only to provide a good source of sustained energy but also to significantly lower blood cholesterol levels.

The health-promoting and anti-ageing effects of eating a wide range of dietary fibre can be summarised as follows:

1 The presence of fibre necessitates more thorough chewing of food and hence slows down eating. It produces a more rapid feeling of 'fullness' and there is less likelihood of overeating and weight gain. Hence eating plenty of fibre is a useful form of calorie control and reduces the risk of obesity.

2 A high proportion of fibre delays the passage of food from the stomach into the intestine so that this becomes a gradual process. This decreases the 'peaking' of blood sugar levels that tends to occur during digestion, resulting in a more sustained provision of energy. Avoidance of blood sugar peaks is important in both the treatment and prevention of diabetes mellitus, one form of which is related to ageing.

3 Dietary fibre promotes the release of pancreatic enzymes and hormones which are vital for digestion and other metabolic processes.

4 Soluble fibre helps to lower blood cholesterol levels. This is important in the prevention of heart and circulatory diseases which are related to ageing.

5 Plenty of fibre ensures the efficient working of the bowel, promoting regularity through absorption of water and providing bulk and weight. This reduces the risk of constipation and the development of diverticulae and haemorrhoids – both conditions that are connected with ageing. Efficient working of the bowel ensures that harmful, anti-oxidant substances that may have been ingested, such as chemical contaminants, are speedily eliminated with faeces.

6 A high proportion of dietary fibre favours the growth of helpful, acid-loving bacteria in the colon at the expense of harmful species that produce

endotoxins. Acid-loving bacteria are able to partially ferment the digested food, providing the body with helpful fatty acids that are utilised by the liver. Energy is also made available to the cells lining the colon. Some of the fatty acids produced, especially butyrate, have been shown to possess anti-carcinogenic properties.

7 Increasing the amount of soluble fibre in the diet is a gentle and helpful form of treatment for irritable bowel syndrome (IBS).

8 Some other forms of fibre, including mucilages (found in seeds and beans), pectins and algal fibre (e.g. agar from certain seaweeds) help to eliminate harmful heavy metal contaminants and other toxins by inhibiting their absorption into the body. This is especially important in view of the fact that these substances are a source of the free radicals that cause harm and age-related damage in the body.

As can be seen, a high fibre diet forms an important part of anti-ageing in the preservation of good health into older age and in the prevention of disease. In general, an adult should try to eat about 30 g (or 10 oz) of fibre each day. This is easily achieved by eating cereals, wholemeal bread, brown rice or pasta, fruits, vegetables and salads. At least five portions of vegetables and fruit each day are considered necessary for good health. Pulses such as lentils, peas and beans are also rich in fibre as well as being a good source of protein.

Some caution may need to be exercised with regard to wheat bran which can be irritant and play a part in food intolerance and allergy. Pure wheat bran, taken in excess, can interfere with the absorption of minerals and vitamins which, in extreme cases, may result in deficiencies. Sufferers from irritable bowel syndrome may need to experiment to find helpful forms of fibre that do not bring on an attack.

Vitamins

Vitamins are a group of organic substances that are required in minute quantities in the diet to maintain good health. They are involved in a large number of metabolic processes, including growth and repair of tissues and organs, utilisation of food and functioning of the immune, nervous, circulatory and hormonal systems.

Vitamins fall into two groups – fat soluble and water soluble. Fat-soluble ones include A, D, E and K. Those that are water-soluble are C (ascorbic acid) and the B group. A lack of a particular vitamin, especially if prolonged, may result in the development of a deficiency disease. Water-soluble vitamins dissolve in water and cannot be stored in the body but must be obtained from the diet on a daily basis. Any excess is simply excreted. Fat-soluble vitamins (with the partial exception of D and K) are also obtained from food but any excess can be stored by the liver. Hence they are needed on a regular basis in order to maintain the body's reserves. However, an excessive intake of some fat-soluble vitamins, especially A and D, (which may result from an overdose of supplements) is dangerous and can have toxic effects due to an accumulation in the liver.

Vitamins are involved in such a wide range of functions that they inevitably have significant anti-ageing properties. Most importantly, some vitamins have direct antioxidant activity, attaching themselves to free radicals and preventing the cellular damage that is believed to be so critical in ageing. In order to fully appreciate the importance of vitamins, it is worth examining them in a little more detail.

Vitamin A

Vitamin A is fat-soluble and plays a vital role in maintaining the health of the epithelial layers of the skin and mucous membranes, so that these function effectively and produce their secretions. These are protective surfaces that form a barrier against potentially harmful particles and substances. Vitamin A has also been shown to enhance the immune response by boosting the cells that fight infections and tumours. It is also needed in the manufacture of rhodopsin or visual purple, a light-sensitive pigment that is essential for vision in dim light. Good sources of vitamin A are orange and yellow vegetables and fruits, particularly carrots, peaches and apricots, and also green vegetables, eggs, full fat dairy products, liver and fish oils.

In fact, the fruits and vegetables just listed contain plant substances called carotenes or carotenoids. Some of these such as beta-carotene, one of the most well-known examples, are precursors of vitamin A, i.e. they are converted into the vitamin within the body. Retinol or vitamin A itself is found in particularly concentrated amounts in liver and fish oils and both it and the carotenoids possess antioxidant and anti-ageing properties.

Deficiency of vitamin A causes a condition known as night blindness as well as a deterioration in the health of mucous membranes. This can cause increased respiratory and ear infections and dry skin, with more susceptibility to skin conditions and dull, lifeless hair. A sustained lack of the vitamin in childhood results in failure to grow and thrive while adults may suffer weight loss and debility. Vitamin A is believed to have anti-cancer properties, possibly helping to protect against cancers of the bowel, bladder, stomach lining and larynx. A good intake of vitamin A (along with C and E) is believed to be important in preventing age-related deterioration in vision. However, as noted above, excessive intake of vitamin A should be avoided, for example you should not take two supplements containing full doses of the vitamin.

Vitamin B$_1$

Vitamin B$_1$ (thiamine or aneurin) is one of the water-soluble group and is involved in carbohydrate metabolism and the vital provision of energy, as well as the healthy functioning of the nervous system and muscles. It plays a part in the mechanisms that combat pain and it may have a role in intellectual functioning. Good sources of B$_1$ are whole grains, potatoes, brown rice, yeast, pulses, green vegetables, eggs, dairy produce, liver, kidney, meat, poultry and fish – a wide range of foods. A slight deficiency causes digestive upset, sickness, constipation, tiredness, irritability and forgetfulness. Prolonged lack of thiamine causes the development of the deficiency disease, beri beri, which occurs mainly in countries in which the staple diet is polished rice. There is inflammation of nerves, fever, breathing difficulties, palpitations and, in severe cases, heart failure and death.

Vitamin B$_2$

Vitamin B$_2$ (riboflavin) is also involved in carbohydrate metabolism (at the level of enzyme reactions in cells) and in the provision of energy. It also helps to maintain the health of the mucous membranes and skin and so is involved in the body's front line defence mechanisms. Like thiamine (B$_1$), it is a water-soluble vitamin and is found in a similar range of foods. A deficiency may cause a sore, irritated tongue and lips, dry skin and scalp and possible nervousness, trembling, giddiness and insomnia.

Vitamin B3

Vitamin B3 (niacin, nicotinic acid) is a water-soluble vitamin involved in the maintenance of healthy blood circulation and also in the functioning of the nervous system and adrenal glands. Good sources include most cereals (excluding maize), nuts, peas, beans, yeast, eggs, dairy produce, dried fruits, globe artichokes, meat, kidney, liver and poultry. A deficiency causes a range of symptoms – sickness, diarrhoea, loss of appetite, peptic ulcer, dermatitis, irritability, depression, tiredness, sleeplessness and depression. In more severe cases, a deficiency disease (pellagra) results in producing the symptoms listed above but with accompanying dementia. Pellagra usually arises in people whose staple diet is maize with an accompanying lack of animal protein and dairy produce.

Vitamin B5

Vitamin B5 (pantothenic acid) is involved in carbohydrate and fat metabolism, the provision of energy, function of the adrenal glands (very important hormone-producing glands) and maintenance of the nervous and immune systems. This water-soluble vitamin is widely found in all types of food and is also produced within the gut. Deficiency is uncommon but low levels may be associated with poor adrenal gland function which, especially at times of stress, may produce symptoms of tiredness, insomnia, headache, sickness and abdominal pains. Low levels of

B_5 may also be implicated in the development of osteoarthritis.

Vitamin B_6

Vitamin B_6 (pyroxidine) is another water-soluble vitamin that is widely found in many foods. It is involved in the metabolism of certain amino acids and in the production of antibodies by the immune system. It also plays a part in carbohydrate and fat metabolism and in the manufacture of red blood cells. A deficiency is uncommon but low levels may be associated with suppression of the immune system and the development of atherosclerosis.

Vitamin B_9

Vitamin B_9 (folic acid) is necessary for the correct functioning of vitamin B_{12} in the production of red blood cells and in the metabolism of carbohydrates, fats and proteins. It is water-soluble and good sources include liver, kidney, green vegetables, yeast, fruits, beans and pulses, whole grains and wheatgerm. A deficiency in folic acid is quite common and produces degrees of anaemia with symptoms of tiredness, insomnia, forgetfulness and irritability. A good intake of folic acid is important for women trying to conceive and for maintaining a healthy pregnancy. Supplements are normally prescribed in these circumstances. A deficiency in folic acid is a common finding in women with cervical dysplasia (abnormality in cells of the cervix which is a precancerous condition) and in those taking oral contraceptives. In addition, it is commonly deficient in people suffering from some forms of mental illness, depression, Crohn's disease and ulcerative colitis. Elderly people are quite commonly found to have low levels of folic acid.

Vitamin B complex

Vitamin B complex (biotin) is a water-soluble vitamin involved in the metabolism of fats, including the production of glucose in conditions in which there is a lack of available carbohydrates. It works in conjunction with insulin, although its mode of operation is independent, and can be important in the treatment of diabetes. Good sources of biotin include egg yolk, liver, kidney, wheat and oats, yeast and nuts. It is also synthesised by gut bacteria. Deficiency is rare in adults but in young infants a lack of biotin may be a cause of cradle cap (seborrhoeic dermatitis).

Vitamin B12

Vitamin B12 (cyanocobalamin, methyl-cobalamin) is necessary for the correct functioning of folic acid. It is also important in the production of genetic material (nucleic acids) and in the maintenance of the fatty, myelin sheaths that surround nerve fibres and are essential for their operation. It is involved in the production of red blood cells, in the metabolism of proteins, carbohydrates and fats and in the maintenance of healthy cells. It is a water-soluble vitamin that is derived from animal sources – egg yolk, dairy produce, meat, liver, kidney and fish but it is often added to (fortified) breakfast cereals. Blood levels of B_{12} are often low in people suffering from Alzheimer's disease and some other forms of psychiatric illnesses. Deficiency results in anaemia but often this is the result of faulty absorption of the vitamin rather than dietary lack. In order for the vitamin to be absorbed, a substance known as intrinsic factor must be produced, along with hydrochloric acid, by secretory cells in the stomach. When this mechanism is defective it may result in the development of pernicious anaemia which is cured by injections of vitamin B_{12} directly into the bloodstream. Dietary deficiency of B_{12}, if prolonged, may result in degeneration of the nervous system producing symptoms of tingling and numbness in the limbs, loss of sensation and some reflexes, lack of coordination, slurring of speech, confusion, irritability and depression. There is also pallor, tiredness, breathlessness and irregular heartbeat caused by the anaemia.

Vitamin B_{12} is believed to have particular anti-ageing properties with regard to the protection of nerve and brain cells from damage by free radicals. Homocysteine is an amino acid that is naturally present in the body. In high concentrations, it is now believed to be a causal factor in heart disease, osteoporosis and arthritis. Vitamin B_{12} is believed to be helpful in neutralising the effects of homocysteine, thus helping to prevent the development of disease. Many researchers believe that eating a diet rich in B_{12} and other B vitamins, including pyroxidine (B_6) and folic acid (B_9), not only protects against heart and circulatory disease but helps to preserve intellectual faculties. The protection is given in at least three ways: by ensuring that the arteries stay healthy so that the brain receives plenty of blood, oxygen and nutrients; by directly influencing the health of nerve cells; and by neutralising the effects of homocysteine.

Vitamin C

Vitamin C (ascorbic acid) is one of the most familiar vitamins whose importance to health has long been recognized. It plays a vital role in the maintenance of cell walls and connective tissue and so is essential for the health of blood vessels, skin, cartilage, tendons, ligaments, gums and lining surfaces. It promotes the uptake and absorption of iron and is critically involved in the effective operation of the immune system, having anti-infection and anti-viral properties. It promotes wound repair and supports the function of the adrenal glands, especially at times of stress. It is involved in the metabolism of fats and in the control of cholesterol and hence plays a significant role in the prevention of atherosclerosis.

Blood levels of vitamin C are often low in people

suffering from asthma, cervical dysplasia (abnormal cells in the cervix or neck of the womb), Crohn's disease, high blood pressure and fistula. Levels of vitamin C in the fluid (aqueous humour) and lens of the human eye are normally high but are low in people with cataracts. Due to its effects on cartilage and connective tissue, lack of the vitamin is thought to be a contributory factor in the development and progression of osteoarthritis. Likewise, vitamin C is vital in preventing gum disease and in the repair of soft tissue injuries.

Vitamin C is unstable and water-soluble, and levels rapidly decline if foods are kept or subjected to heat, light and cooking. The best sources are fresh fruits (especially citrus fruits, black and red berries, currants, grapes, kiwis, paw paws, peaches, nectarines and mangoes) and vegetables (e.g. potatoes, tomatoes, green, leafy vegetables, Brussels sprouts, red peppers). A prolonged and severe deficiency of vitamin C causes the development of scurvy, the symptoms of which include bleeding gums, loosened teeth, bleeding beneath the skin and into joints, ulcers, anaemia, tiredness, confusion, loss of muscle mass and strength, and diarrhoea. Eventually, the major organs are affected and death results – a common outcome in the early days of long sea voyages aboard sailing ships. Severe scurvy is rare but some symptoms of deficiency are occasionally reported in those whose dietary intake is very low.

Vitamin C is known to have vital antioxidant properties, combating the free radicals that are involved in the ageing process. It is present in high quantities in foods that are protective against certain cancers, heart disease and some other conditions. Some people take large doses of the vitamin, believing that this protects them against catching the common cold, although this has not been scientifically proved. Excess vitamin C is excreted and there is evidence that high doses in supplement form can cause some harm in susceptible people. Eating plenty of the foods that contain high levels of vitamin C is a different matter and forms an important part of both healthy eating and adopting an anti-ageing plan.

Vitamin D

Vitamin D is a fat-soluble vitamin which, in the form of cholecalciferol, is produced within the body by the action of sunlight on the skin. Vitamin D is vital in the control of blood calcium levels, promoting an increased absorption of the mineral from the intestine so that there is a good supply for the production and repair of bones and teeth. Vitamin D also promotes the uptake of the mineral phosphorus, which is equally important in the health of bones, teeth and muscles. Good dietary sources of the vitamin are oily fish such as mackerel, sardines, salmon, tuna, kippers and herring, egg yolk, liver, full fat dairy produce, evaporated milk and fortified foods, especially margarine and breakfast cereals.

Vitamin D is converted by the liver into a more potent form and it appears that in some cases it is this mechanism that is at fault rather than dietary deficiency. Levels are often low in people who suffer from Crohn's disease and ulcerative colitis and also among ethnic communities who may cover up completely in the sun and eat a diet that lacks adequate vitamin D. A slight deficiency causes tooth decay, softening of the bones, muscular cramps and weakness. Severe and prolonged deficiency results in rickets in children and osteomalacia in adults. These conditions are characterised by soft bones that bend out of shape causing deformity and risk of fractures. It is not advisable to take supplements of vitamin D on its own as this is one of the vitamins that has toxic effects in large doses. People with normal exposure to the sun manufacture enough storable vitamin D to last them for one year and also obtain 'top-ups' from food.

Vitamin E

Vitamin E consists of a group of fat-soluble compounds called tocopherols which are widely found in a range of foods. Good dietary sources include nuts and seeds, vegetable oils, green vegetables, eggs, wholegrains and cereals, pulses, soya products and margarine. Vitamin E is involved in maintaining the health of red blood cells and cell membranes, in resisting infection and plays a part in blood clotting. It has proven antioxidant activity and is believed to be protective in atherosclerosis, some cancers, stroke and heart disease. Deficiency is rare but may cause unhealthy skin and hair and be a contributory factor in some miscarriages and some cases of male prostate gland enlargement.

Anti-ageing experts consider vitamin E to be one of the most important micronutrients and generally recommend supplements in addition to eating foods which are naturally rich in the vitamin.

Vitamin K
Vitamin K (menadione) is fat-soluble and is essential for the clotting of blood. It is manufactured by bacteria naturally present in the large intestine. It is also found in liver, kidney, green vegetables such as broccoli, spinach and Brussels sprouts, seaweed, wheatgerm and eggs. Deficiency is rare in healthy persons but has been reported in those suffering from ulcerative colitis and Crohn's disease. It may rarely occur if large and prolonged doses of antibiotics have to be taken as these may disrupt the natural bacterial balance in the gut. Symptoms include nosebleeds and subcutaneous bleeding.

Some anti-ageing experts believe that vitamin K is more important than is currently recognized in preventing age-related effects and recommend the use of supplements.

Vitamin summary
It can be seen that most vitamins have numerous func-

tions that are essential for the maintenance of good health and for the prevention of disease. Many of the functions in which they are involved are connected with the processes of anti-ageing and a good dietary intake of vitamins is essential at every age to safeguard health. The vitamins that are considered to be the most important in anti-ageing are B_{12}, C, E and K. For healthy people, nutritionists usually recommend fulfilling vitamin needs from food and, perhaps not surprisingly, evidence suggests that this is the most effective way for the human body. However, there are many circumstances in which supplements are useful and might be recommended, e.g. during periods of illness or convalescence and in older age, when absorption of nutrients from the gut is compromised. Anti-ageing specialists are more likely to advocate the use of vitamin supplements, particularly the ones listed above, for their particular benefits in combating age-related effects.

Minerals

Minerals are found in rocks and metals but are also present in all living things and play a vital part in many metabolic processes. Some minerals, notably calcium and phosphorus, are present in significant amounts in the human body, mainly in bones and teeth. Others, for example iron, iodine and sodium, occur in extremely small quantities but are essential substances for health. Minerals that are needed only in minute amounts are called *trace elements*. As with vitamins, a lack of a particular mineral can lead to a deficiency disease with the appearance of a set of symptoms that may develop over a long period of time. The effects of deficiency may be quite complex in some cases and may arise either as a direct result of dietary insufficiency or because of malabsorption of the mineral or some other dysfunction within the body.

As noted above, minerals are involved in very many metabolic processes, including those that combat illness and the effects of ageing. Some have direct anti-oxidant effects while others work indirectly, being necessary for the function of vitamins, enzymes and hormones. The importance of minerals has been increasingly recognized by health specialists in recent years but their critical role is probably less fully appreciated than that of vitamins. Hence it is worth examining the role of minerals in a little more detail.

Sodium
Sodium, obtained from the diet in the form of common salt (sodium chloride) is essential in minute quantities for the correct functioning of nerves and as a vital constituent of cellular and tissue fluids. The amount needed is readily obtained from natural foods, most of which contain traces of salt without the need for further addition. The problem for people eating a western diet, which relies heavily on processed

foods that contain a lot of added salt, is an excessive intake that can contribute towards a number of serious health problems. Included in their number are heart and circulatory disease, high blood pressure and kidney disorders. These disorders are often age-related and it is important to realize that one risk factor implicated in their development can easily be eliminated, simply by not adding salt to food during cooking or at the table. Also, by avoiding eating too many processed foods, or at least choosing reduced salt varieties and checking labels, intake can be further controlled. Many people (and animals also) enjoy the taste of salt which can enhance the flavour of food and may act as a preservative. However, the taste for salt is an acquired habit and one that, with a little perseverance, can be broken. Using dried or fresh herbs as a substitute for salt adds interest to cooking and many of these have beneficial antioxidant and anti-ageing properties (*see* herbal remedies, page 179). In the event of a salty meal being eaten, several glasses of water should be drunk to dilute the effects and ease the strain on the kidneys.

Potassium

Potassium is a vital component of cell and tissue fluids, helping to maintain the electrolyte-water balance and also essential for nerve function. The balance between potassium and sodium levels in the body may be quite significant in the development of some diseases and conditions. For example, low potassium/ high sodium ratios are a factor in the development of high blood pressure and stress. A deficiency in potassium causes appetite loss and sickness, bloating, muscle weakness, thirst and 'pins and needles' sensations. Blood pressure falls may lead to light-headedness and in very severe, rare cases, unconsciousness and coma. A normal, varied diet should contain sufficient potassium although levels are often low in highly processed foods.

Calcium

Calcium is present in significant amounts in the human body, forming about 2% of the total mass and overwhelmingly concentrated in the bones and teeth. Calcium is essential for the growth and repair of the skeleton and teeth and it is particularly important for growing children and pregnant, menopausal and postmenopausal women to ensure that they have a good dietary intake of the mineral.

The uptake and utilisation of calcium is controlled by vitamin D but the mineral must first be broken down by stomach acid into a form that can be used. The situation can be quite complicated with regard to the development and progression of conditions relating to calcium and there may not be a straightforward relationship with dietary intake of the mineral. For example, osteoporosis patients are quite frequently found to have low levels of stomach acid and the most potent form of vitamin D rather than a dietary lack of calcium. Likewise, people suffering from Crohn's disease or irritable bowel syndrome may go short of calcium as a result of deficiency of vitamin D, rather than a lack of the mineral. However, on the other hand, some people with high blood pressure have been shown to have a low dietary intake of calcium. A deficiency in calcium, which is uncommon in those who are in good health and who eat a normal varied diet, causes rickets in children and osteomalacia in adults (*see* vitamin D, page 76).

Calcium-rich foods include milk and dairy products, fish, flour, bread and fortified cereals. Due to its vital role in maintaining the health of the bones, anti-ageing specialists recommend calcium supplements for older women and those at risk of osteoporosis.

Iron

Iron is an essential component of haemoglobin, the respiratory compound in red blood cells that transports oxygen from the lungs to the tissues and carbon dioxide in the opposite direction. Iron-rich foods include red meat, liver, kidney, egg yolk, cocoa, nuts, green vegetables, especially spinach, dried fruits, pulses, fortified flour and cereals. Iron is more easily absorbed from meat but its uptake is also enhanced by eating plenty of vitamin C. A deficiency in iron causes anaemia, producing symptoms of tiredness, shortness of breath, feeling cold, dizziness, pallor and possible swelling of the ankles, weight loss and irregular heart-beat. However, several medical conditions and illnesses can also result in anaemia which is not produced by a dietary lack of iron. Slight anaemia is quite common, especially among women, and may not necessarily be noticed. Whatever the cause, iron supplements are usually prescribed for anyone medically diagnosed with anaemia and the mineral is also routinely given to pregnant women and those who have just given birth. Anti-ageing experts believe that iron supplements should be avoided unless they have been prescribed for sound medical reasons. It is believed that excess iron in the blood (obtained from supplements rather than food) may favour attacks by free radicals and so enhance the processes of ageing.

Phosphorus

Phosphorus is present in the body in considerable amounts, accounting for about 1% of total weight and concentrated in the bones and teeth, in which it plays a vital role in growth, repair and maintenance. Phosphorus is also essential in energy metabolism and muscular activity and in the function of certain enzymes. It affects the absorption of other elements and compounds from the small intestine and the body's supply is totally renewed every two to three years. A deficiency in phosphorus is unlikely in those eating a normal, varied diet since it is widely found in foods but is especially concentrated in animal products. In fact, in western countries, the opposite problem of excess intake of the mineral is more likely to occur due to a high consumption of meat and dairy produce at the expense of plant-based foods. An elevated intake of phosphorus can reduce or prevent the absorption of iron, calcium, zinc and magnesium and may be a factor in the incidence of osteoporosis and a number of other disorders. Following guidelines for healthy eating should ensure that intake of phosphorus is adequate rather than excessive and supplements are not usually recommended.

Magnesium

Magnesium is required for the growth, repair and maintenance of bones and teeth, the effective functioning of nerves and muscles, and for metabolic processes involving certain enzymes. It also has a role in the functioning of vitamins B_1 and B_{12}. Magnesium is widely found in many foods, including green vegetables, cereals, whole grains, meat, milk and dairy produce, eggs, shellfish, nuts and pulses. Deficiency (which should normally be unlikely in those eating a varied diet), causes anxiety, insomnia, cramps, trembling, palpitations and loss of appetite and weight. Low levels of magnesium may possibly be indicated in a number of diseases and conditions including high blood pressure and osteoporosis. Anti-ageing specialists may recommend magnesium supplements as part of a treatment plan for the control of these conditions.

Iodine

Iodine is vital for the correct functioning of the thyroid gland and is present in two thyroid hormones that are essential for the regulation of metabolism and growth. It is present in high quantities in seaweed, seafoods, and vegetables and fruits grown on iodine-rich soil. Likewise, animals which have grazed on grass growing on iodine-rich soils incorporate the mineral into their muscle (meat).

Deficiency is relatively rare because iodine is added to table and cooking salt and is present in staple foods such as bread and cereals. If it does occur, it results in goitre, where the thyroid gland enlarges, producing a lump in the neck and causing symptoms of tiredness, lowered metabolism, weakness and weight gain. Iodine deficiency combined with hypothyroidism may be associated with fibrocystic diseases of the breasts and some cases of breast cancer. Supplements are not regarded as necessary except under medical advice.

Manganese

Manganese is essential for the activity of many enzymes and metabolic reactions. It is also involved in nerve and muscle function and in growth and repair of the skeleton. It is a co-factor in a vital enzyme of glucose metabolism, and some people with diabetes mellitus and rheumatoid arthritis have been shown to be deficient in the mineral. It is necessary for the activity of an enzyme called (manganese) superoxide dismutase (SOD) which has important antioxidant activity and is available in supplement form. Manganese is widely found in many foods but especially in whole grains, nuts, cereals, avocado pears, pulses and tea and deficiency is normally rare. Supplements of manganese are not recommended as an excess of the mineral can be harmful, causing learning disabilities and central nervous system effects.

Copper

Copper is involved in the activity of many enzymes and metabolic functions and in the production of red blood cells and connective tissue. It is necessary for bone growth and repair and is involved in the metabolism of fats. The zinc-copper balance has been shown to be important in the development of some conditions as the two minerals may 'compete' with one another to a certain extent. A deficiency is uncommon but may be a factor in the development of two age-related conditions, atherosclerosis and osteoarthritis. Deficiency reduces the number of white blood cells, hence lowering immunity, may cause diarrhoea and produces changes in the hair. The mineral is widely found in many foods but especially rich sources are shellfish, nuts, liver, kidney and cocoa. Copper supplements are not recommended. An excess can be harmful and may be involved in causing joint damage, learning difficulties and in increased susceptibility to gum disease. However, the wearing of copper bracelets can be helpful for some people suffering from rheumatoid arthritis.

Chromium

Chromium is important in a range of metabolic activities, particularly the utilisation and storage of sugars and fats. It is involved in the activity of insulin, in glucose tolerance in diabetes and in immune system function. Chromium is also necessary for the correct functioning of the voluntary muscles that move the bones and joints.

Chromium is found in whole and unrefined foods, including wholemeal flour, whole grains, cereals, brewer's yeast, nuts, meat, liver, kidney, vegetables, mushrooms and fresh fruits. Levels in the body naturally decline with age and some researchers believe that this may be implicated in maturity-onset diabetes and in ageing processes connected with declining immunity. A deficiency in the mineral may cause irritability and depression, forgetfulness and sleep disturbances. Chromium is available in supplement form and may be recommended by anti-ageing specialists. However, people who are diabetic should not use this (or any other supplement) without seeking medical advice.

Sulphur

Sulphur is involved in amino acid metabolism and

the manufacture of proteins and hence is important in the structural components of the body – bones, teeth, nails and skin. The sulphur-containing amino acids, methionine and cysteine are believed to be involved in human longevity (*see* glutathione, SAMe below) and levels of these natural anti-ageing substances tend to decline in older age. A deficiency of sulphur is not normally found. Good dietary sources are eggs, meat, liver, pulses, garlic, onions, nuts, brewer's yeast, fish and dairy produce.

Strontium

Strontium is similar in composition to calcium and, like that mineral, is found concentrated in bones and teeth. Strontium is naturally found in milk and dairy products and helps to ensure the strength of bone. It can also be beneficial in the treatment of osteoporosis.

Boron

Boron is thought to be involved in the utilisation of calcium and in the activity of vitamin D and oestrogen. It is thought to be necessary for the conversion of vitamin D into its most potent, active form which occurs within the kidneys. Good sources of the mineral are fresh vegetables and fruits. It can be beneficial in the treatment of osteoporosis. Supplements are not normally recommended since the mineral can be toxic in high doses.

Selenium

Selenium is a mineral that has come to be well known in recent years for its powerful antioxidant activity, especially when combined with vitamin E. Selenium is the co-factor necessary for the activity of the enzyme glutathione peroxidase which mops up free radicals. It is also involved in immune system function, reducing the formation of certain prostaglandins (hormone-like chemicals) and leukotrienes (compounds in white blood cells) that are involved in inflammatory and allergic responses. Selenium also supports the correct functioning of the liver. It is estimated that many people have a dietary insufficiency of this important, anti-ageing mineral. Good sources are brazil nuts, whole grains and cereals, shellfish, halibut, tuna, egg yolks, kidney, liver, garlic, radishes and yeast. As a supplement, selenium along with vitamin E can be beneficial in the treatment of various disorders including acne, psoriasis, cervical dysplasia (pre-cancer of the cervix), skin cancer, rheumatoid arthritis, soft tissue injuries and gum disease. It is also believed to be protective and helpful in the prevention and treatment of heart disease, and deficiency can have effects upon the heart and circulation. It is widely available as a supplement and is one of the most useful weapons in the anti-ageing armoury.

Zinc

Zinc is essential for the functioning of numerous enzymes

and is widely involved in metabolic processes. It is necessary for the utilisation of vitamin A and vital in immune system functioning. It is an antiviral agent, is involved in the healing of wounds and has important antioxidant activity. It has an essential role in insulin metabolism and the control of blood sugar levels. Deficiency has wide-ranging effects including poor growth and physical development, and retardation of intellectual faculties, as well as slow wound healing. Deficiency is common in people suffering from medical conditions such as Crohn's disease, gum disease and hypothyroidism. It is believed to be implicated in susceptibility to viral infections and possibly in the development of diabetes mellitus. Zinc is widely found in many foods but especially good sources are shellfish, particularly oysters, egg yolk, liver, meat, whole grains and cereals, whole meal flour, seeds and nuts. It is available in supplement form and is one of the products that may be recommended by anti-ageing specialists.

Minerals summary

It can be seen that vitamins and minerals have very wide-ranging activities within the human body which involve complex interactions, the ramifications of which are not yet fully understood in all cases. They are important both in the maintenance of good health and in combating age-related conditions and effects. It is interesting to note that they are widely found in a variety of natural foods of both plant and animal origin.

Recent surveys have suggested that vegetarians live, on average, for one year longer than those who eat meat and fish but the true picture may be more complex than it first appears. So much depends upon what the groups of people who have been studied actually *are* eating and with what frequency. The evidence for the health (and longevity) benefits of, for example, fish oils is overwhelming and, as can be seen from these pages, it cannot be denied that lean, red meat contains useful vitamins, minerals and protein.

It would be interesting to know whether the surveys have compared people who eat a lot of meat (and hence cholesterol), perhaps at the expense of plenty of fruit and vegetables, with those who are true vegetarians. Or, have they compared non-vegetarians eating a healthy, anti-ageing diet that is largely plant/wholefood based but includes oily fish, chicken and a sparse consumption of lean meat, with vegetarians? The latter would give a more accurate picture of the true situation with regard to longevity and vegetarianism, and is perhaps the sort of study that needs to be carried out in the future. Evidence (from the pattern of teeth) suggests that human beings evolved as omnivores and a diet that contains fish and chicken as well as plenty of vegetables, fruits, grains, nuts, seeds and pulses is consistent with both healthy eating and anti-ageing.

Super substances

Some experts believe that there are a group of 'super' substances that are especially effective in counteracting the effects of ageing and so are worthy of special mention. New substances are being researched and studied and there may well be others that will be included in this elite group in the future. But the following are the ones to pay special attention to if you are interested in anti-ageing!

Carotenes

Carotenes are naturally-occurring, organic substances containing carotenoids, the orange, yellow or red pigments that are quite widely found in plant and some animal tissues (e.g. egg yolk, milk fat). About 40 to 50 of the carotenoids that have been studied can be converted into vitamin A and are precursors of provitamin A. Also, many carotenes, of which the best known example is beta-carotene, have been demonstrated to have potent antioxidant activity. Carotenes are naturally deposited in body tissues and in the thymus gland which, as we have seen, is an important organ of the immune system. There exists a growing body of evidence suggesting that the concentration of carotenes within the body, along with naturally occurring antioxidant enzymes, are factors determining the length of lifespan in mammals, including human beings. It is known that the levels of these protective substances naturally decline with age, but perhaps those who are long-lived maintain higher concentrations in their tissues than those who are not. It has been demonstrated that eating a diet rich in carotenes raises the level of these nutrients in the tissues, hence increasing antioxidant availability. The best sources are carrots, green leafy vegetables such as broccoli and spinach, beets, sweet potatoes (yams), squashes, pumpkins and coloured vegetables. A good intake of carotenes helps to protect the body against certain forms of cancer and supports the immune system in its fight against infection (*see also* Free radicals and antioxidants in Why Do We Age?, page 17).

Flavonoids

Flavonoids are a group of naturally occurring plant pigments that are widely found in fruits and green vegetables. They are the most potent known antioxidants, having the ability to counteract free radicals, but they also appear to have other anti-ageing properties as well. Flavonoids appear to have anti-cancer, anti-viral, anti-allergy and anti-inflammatory properties and some also have hormonal-type activity. They are protective of the heart, circulation and skin. It has been discovered that some flavonoids appear to possess particular affinity for certain tissues. Several thousand flavonoids have been identified and studied, particularly those from plants and herbs that have a long history of traditional medicinal use and their effectiveness is tending to be proved rather than disproved by scientific scrutiny.

Flavonoids form a very broad group of substances that have wide-ranging effects. Particularly important are the anthocyanidins found in highly coloured berries, especially cranberries, bilberries, cherries, blackcurrants, strawberries, raspberries and grapes. Anti-ageing specialists recommend that these fruits are eaten as frequently as possible – at least once each week. Isoflavones are another important group, some of which have natural hormonal activity. Apart from the fruits mentioned above, rich sources of flavonoids include green vegetables such as broccoli, citrus fruit, apples, mangoes, pomegranates, seeds, tomatoes (including cooked and concentrated forms as in tomato sauce), herbs, e.g. thyme, marjoram, basil, oregano, garlic, onions. Also, red wine (but no more than two small glasses each day), tea and green tea, fruit juices (cranberry and grape), soya milk and soya bean products.

It can be seen that eating a diet rich in fruit and vegetables is important not only to supply vitamins, minerals and fibre but also to protect the body against disease and ageing effects as well.

Glutathione

Glutathione is a naturally occurring antioxidant, synthesized within the body from certain amino acids, that has attracted particular attention from specialists in ageing. This is due to the fact that while levels are normally low in the elderly and those who are chronically sick, those who are long-lived maintain a higher concentration of this substance in their blood. Glutathione is available as a supplement but good natural sources are, once again, fresh vegetables and fruit, although it is easily destroyed by cooking. Carrots, tomatoes, broccoli, potatoes, spinach, asparagus, avocado pears, water melon and red meat are all particularly useful sources.

Co-enzyme Q10

Co-enzyme Q10 is a naturally occurring antioxidant enzyme that is found in almost all human cells and tissues and plays a vital role in energy metabolism. Levels begin to decline in middle age and it is believed that it may help to protect the heart and immune system. Good sources of this substance are oily fish (e.g. mackerel, sardines, herring, tuna, salmon, trout), nuts (e.g. walnuts, almonds, Brazil nuts), soya beans, soya products and green vegetables, especially spinach. It is also available as a supplement and one that is becoming increasingly popular in preventing age-related conditions.

Carnosine

Carnosine is a dipeptide (protein) compound, composed of two amino acid molecules, with the chemical name beta-ananyl-L-histidine. It occurs naturally in muscles, the brain and nerves and in the lens of the eye and, as one of the most interesting and exciting substances in the field of anti-ageing, it is worthy of special mention. It is true to say that its potential is only just beginning to be realized. Although carnosine has been known for many years, it is only recently that scientific studies have started to reveal its incredible properties.

Carnosine is a potent antioxidant that seems to boost activity against free radicals in a number of different organs, including the brain, heart, stomach and liver. It has important effects in the muscles and during hard exercise, slows up the build-up of lactic acid and enables the muscles to work for longer without becoming fatigued. Its antioxidant properties are especially important in this situation since exercise produces free radicals through oxidation. Carnosine boosts the immune system by increasing the longevity of neutrophils (white blood cells which consume bacteria) and hence is involved in the fight against infection. It also promotes the secretion of chemical substances called interleukins which are directly involved in the immune response. It has also been shown to promote wound healing.

In Alzheimer's disease, there is a build-up of 'plaques' of unnatural, damaged material damage in the brains of patients. One of the substances responsible for this cellular damage is beta-amyloid. Carnosine appears to have a protective effect, helping to block the action of beta-amyloid and there is growing interest in its potential in the prevention and treatment of dementia.

As a result of normal metabolism, a process called glycosylation occurs which involves sugar aldehyde molecules reacting with the amino acids of proteins. This results in the creation of abnormal and ineffective cross-linked proteins and the production of damaging Advance Glycosylation End products or AGEs. The proteins that are damaged include vital molecules such as enzymes and DNA. In younger people, AGEs are quickly eliminated but it is thought that this process is less effective as ageing progresses. The build-up of AGEs and cross-linked proteins is believed to be responsible for many age-related conditions. These include some cancers, arterial disease, diabetes, cataracts, kidney disease, immune system disorders, skin conditions, nerve damage, Alzheimer's disease and abnormal blood clotting. Carnosine inactivates some of the biochemical pathways that cause cross-linking and the production of AGEs, thus helping to protect the body against their damaging effects. It is also active against some other toxic, damaging substances such as aldehyde, and is able to chelate poisonous metallic ions. Chelation is a reaction which involves an organic molecule (in this case, carnosine) joining onto an unwanted toxic metal ion to produce a harmless, closed ring compound that can be eliminated from the body.

In laboratory experiments, cultures of human fibroblasts (a type of cell found in connective tissue) were treated with carnosine and it was found that this increased their 'life expectancy' by 20%. This meant that the cells continued to divide and function beyond the point when they would normally have died. If it acts in this way on all body cells, carnosine may indeed be able to promote longevity. Carnosine has already been used successfully (in eye drops) to treat glaucoma and it may well prove useful in the prevention and treatment of cataract and other age-related eye conditions.

Carnosine is manufactured as a supplement but it is not yet widely used or well-known. Some anti-ageing specialists believe that it is set to become one of the key products in promoting a long, healthy and active life because of its multi-action capabilities. Good dietary sources of carnosine are poultry and lean red meat. If you are not a vegetarian it may make sense to at least eat plenty of the former until supplements become more readily available.

Phospholipids

Phospholipids – lecithin (phosphatidyl choline and phosphatidyl serine – are naturally occurring, organic substances containing two fatty acids and phosphate, that possess both water-attracting and water-repelling properties. Due to this latter property, phospholipids readily form membrane-like structures and as bi-layers, or double layers, they form an important constituent of animal and plant cell membranes. One of the best known phospholipids is lecithin which is readily found in the membranes of living cells. It is also a component of bile (a digestive fluid) and acts as a surfactant in the lungs, reducing surface tension. Lecithin, and its equivalent, phosphatidyl choline, have beneficial effects on the brain, nervous system and skin, in the absorption of some vitamins and in the control of blood cholesterol. Good sources include soya beans, corn, walnuts, wholewheat, wheatgerm, egg yolks and liver. It is also available as a dietary supplement and the most useful types to take should contain at least 30% phosphatidyl choline.

Phosphatidyl serine (PS) is a related, naturally occurring phospholipid that, in scientific trials, has been found to have positive effects on the memory and mental capabilities. Soya beans and produce made from them contain some PS but the best sources are animal brains. Of course, these no longer feature in the national diet and, post-BSE, brains are unlikely to make a comeback! However, PS is available as a supplement that is prepared from soya beans and can be taken to improve memory and intellectual faculties.

Alpha lipoic acid

Alpha lipoic acid or ALA is a naturally occurring, vitamin-like substance that is manufactured within the body. It has two essential roles within the body; firstly, it is a vital coenzyme in the cycle of biochemical reactions that provide energy to all cells. Secondly, it is a potent antioxidant that is unique in that it is both water and fat soluble (compare with other vitamins) and so has wide-ranging activity within the body. Not only is it a powerful antioxidant in its own right, it also possesses the ability to revitalize other antioxidants including forms of vitamin C, vitamin E, coenzyme Q10 and glutathione.

Alpha lipoic acid has been used for many years to treat adult onset diabetes. But it has also been found useful in the treatment of cirrhosis of the liver, cataracts, glaucoma, heart disease, nerve damage and heavy metal poisoning. It has been shown to be supportive of the liver, being able to help detoxification, especially of heavy and toxic metals. More recently, ALA has been shown to be helpful in the treatment of HIV infections and AIDS.

It is believed that the body manufactures enough ALA for normal purposes but that during ageing or in the event of disease, the amount is insufficient for the amount of damage that is sustained. ALA is found in red meat, liver, potatoes and brewer's yeast but it is usually taken in supplement form. As such, it has a long history of use and is considered to be very safe, producing no significant side effect. Supplementation may, however, interfere with the natural utilisation of certain vitamins if particular conditions apply.

Hence supplements of ALA are not recommended except under medical advice.

Food is the best medicine

It is hoped that these pages have helped the reader to understand just how important food is in achieving good health and supporting the processes of anti-ageing. We all have to eat and most people in the UK are in the fortunate position of being able to make choices in their diet. Most nutritionists believe that the best way to obtain the helpful, anti-ageing substances that we have discussed is through the food that we eat – something that is available to all. Anti-ageing experts certainly advocate the use of supplements but some of these, as we have seen, are also available in food. Supplements can, in any event, be expensive but by choosing the most helpful diet at every age, you can reduce your need for them, enabling you to use only those that are most beneficial and, hopefully, affordable.

Water of life

Before leaving the subject of diet, it is helpful to look at the essential role played by water in the maintenance of good health and in the prevention of certain age-related conditions. It can be difficult to accept that in common with all living organisms, human beings are largely composed of water. In fact, the human body is made up of about 60% water that must be continuously replenished as it is constantly being lost. Water is naturally eliminated through respiration, sweating and urination with more being lost during hot weather. It is an essential component of tissue, lubricating fluids and blood, and is necessary for most body processes including digestion and elimination of waste. An average adult person requires about three litres of water each day, depending upon body size and weight. Most of this (62%) needs to be taken in as fluid while the remainder is supplied from the water content in foods, with a small amount generated by metabolic processes.

Water is essential to life and this is emphasized by the fact that while we can survive for perhaps two or three weeks without food, we die within a matter of days without water. Health experts recommend drinking six to eight glasses of plain water each day, along with other drinks. It is estimated that many people do not drink the necessary amount of fluid and are, as a consequence, slightly dehydrated most of the time. This can cause symptoms of headache, irritability and forgetfulness and puts a strain on the kidneys. Particular care must be taken in older age as it seems that the sensation of feeling thirsty does not work as effectively as in youth. Hence many older people may become slightly dehydrated through not drinking enough due to lack of thirst. Drinking plenty of plain water helps to reduce the risk of kidney stones and urinary tract infections. In the event of an infection occurring (something that many women experience at some stage in life), drinking plenty of water helps to flush out the causative organisms. Everyone should drink more water during hot weather to compensate for the increased loss due to sweating. Drinking plenty of water, especially in frequent, small mouthfuls, is particularly important for anyone suffering from a stomach bug, as diarrhoea and vomiting are other common causes of dehydration.

Exercise

WE NOW turn to the second area of life over which we all have indiv idual control and which, used wisely, helps to ensure that we will live a long, healthy and active life. There is universal agreement among health professionals about the benefits of regular exercise and anti-ageing specialists are no exception. However, they may recommend certain forms of exercise as being particularly beneficial at different ages in life.

Regular physical exercise is vital throughout life to help maintain good health. It helps to burn up any extra calories taken in as food and so reduces the likelihood of these being converted into fat. Exercise trains the heart so that its muscle fibres become stronger and it is able to pump a greater volume of blood with each beat, hence making the circulation more efficient. This is achieved by fairly vigorous, regular (aerobic) exercise, sufficient to raise the heart and respiration rate, which is initially carried out for about 20 minutes three times a week. This can be increased, if desired, as fitness improves. Types of exercise include brisk walking, cycling, dancing, sports, etc., and it is best if these become a regular part of young adult life and are then continued with, at a less vigorous level, in middle and older age. This type of exercise confers many health benefits. The resting heartbeat rate slows down and the circulation is more efficient, blood pressure is lowered and basal metabolic rate is raised. This means that the body uses more calories even while at rest, hence lessening the likelihood of weight gain.

Other forms of exercise, particularly weight-bearing activities, pump calcium into the bones and help to maintain their density and strength. This has been shown to be particularly beneficial for those in middle and older age, as it significantly reduces the rate at which bone density declines, lessening the risk of fractures associated with osteoporosis. Last, but by no means least, exercise confers a sense of well-being and promotes restful sleep and a healthy appetite. Many people have heard about the 'exercise high' experienced by athletes that is believed to be caused by a release in the brain of natural opiate-like chemicals called endorphins. However, you do not have to be a supreme athlete to experience the 'feel good' factor associated with exercise. For all people, even those suffering from some chronic disabilities and disorders, exercise within the limits of their strength helps to make them feel better, and it is worth remembering that exercise is recommended in the treatment of depression.

Another benefit, and perhaps one that is not mentioned as often as it should be, is that exercise activities can be a route to self-discovery. There are very many people who have one day decided to have a try at some activity, perhaps at the persuasion of family or friends and against their better judgement, not expecting to enjoy it at all, only to find themselves 'hooked'. It is also the case that many exercise activities lead to the formation of new friendships and an expansion of one's social life. As we shall see later, these psychological factors have an important part to play in anti-ageing. Some Far Eastern exercise disciplines perfectly combine these physical, psychological and spiritual factors and are highly beneficial for those following an anti-ageing lifestyle.

In summary, different forms of exercise and activity have beneficial effects upon both physical and psychological health, helping to maintain a fit, active body and mind. Bodily health is improved by exercise in three main ways.

Fitness, stamina and endurance

Fitness, stamina and endurance are required to sustain a period of vigorous activity without having to stop because your heart is racing and you are gasping for breath. This must be built up gradually by an exercise regime that steadily improves the heart, circulation, lungs and respiration, beginning with short periods of fairly vigorous activity of about 15 or 20 minutes, three times a week. An improvement in fitness is usually noticed quite quickly, after about three weeks of training when the person starts to find that the exercise is easier to carry out than before. The time period can then be increased or the exercise carried out more frequently. Brisk walking, jogging, cycling, dancing, vigorous swimming, many sports and various 'everyday' activities involving physical labour will all improve fitness.

Flexibility

Flexibility is the ability of joints and muscles to perform their full range of movements – flexing and straightening, stretching, rotating and twisting – with suppleness and ease and with no resistance or discomfort. There are very many forms of exercise that fulfil this function, including some of the Oriental disciplines. Bending, stretching and general 'loosening up' should be performed before and after taking part in more vigorous activities and sports to lessen the risk of injuries or cramp. Exercises in this category are also an ideal choice for older people.

Toning

Toning and firming up of the body's musculature, leading to an overall increase in muscle bulk and an improvement in posture, is achieved by the performance of strength exercises and the use of weights.

The exercises and activities mentioned above also play a part in this and the importance of weight bearing to maintain the strength of bones has already been noted. However, certain medial conditions preclude the use of weights and it is essential to proceed cautiously, with proper supervision and advice, especially when using gym equipment.

Beginning an exercise routine

It is advisable for any person aged over 35 years or anyone who is overweight or who has previously been inactive to have a medical check-up before taking up any form of vigorous physical activity. Also, older people or those with a known condition or disability should always check with their doctor to make sure that the exercise is suitable for them. A great deal depends upon your existing physical health and condition, whatever age you are, and so the golden rule is to be honest with yourself and to apply plain common sense! It is no use booking the squash court if you have previously been a couch potato but if, on the other hand, you are a fit 70-year-old who enjoys hill walking, you are unlikely to need a medical check-up before going on a Sunday afternoon stroll!

Do not exercise immediately after eating a substantial meal. It is best to eat a starchy meal, which will provide plenty of energy, about three hours before beginning the activity and to drink plenty of water both before, during and after exercising. Do not exercise if you are feverish or unwell in any way as this simply puts a strain on the system, hinders recovery and can be dangerous. Listen to your body and stop if something becomes uncomfortable or painful or if you are fighting for breath – it means that you are trying to do too much too soon.

Always make sure that you are wearing the correct clothing, footwear and headgear appropriate for the activity and that it is of good quality and fits well. Injuries are often caused through neglect in this area and the cost of equipment is a factor that must be considered before embarking upon a new form of exercise or activity. However, remember that exercising for health and anti-ageing can be undertaken very easily and cheaply and so there are no excuses not to get started!

Fitting exercise in

Most people recognize the need to undertake physical exercise but for many, a perceived lack of free times makes it difficult for them to fit this into their daily routine. Also, some people (especially men), make the mistake of launching into some fast and vigorous form of exercise straight away, without taking the time and trouble to first build up their fitness. This can be dangerous if there is any underlying undiagnosed condition such as heart disease and may easily cause soft tissue injuries when muscles and joints are suddenly put under unaccustomed stress. It is also unsatisfactory, since a person who does this is likely to fail at the activity in the first instance, and may easily become discouraged and lapse back into taking little or no exercise at all. So, as we have seen, another important rule is be prepared to proceed slowly and take pleasure in the small improvements that you *will* notice in your health as you exercise. The good news in this respect, and one that many people fail to realize, is how much of a difference can be made by just small adjustments in daily routine and lifestyle.

People who are prepared to take a critical look at this usually find that there are places where they can fit in some physical exercise without unduly disrupting their schedule. A good and much quoted example of this is to use the stairs, rather than the lift at work or park the car further away in order to fit in a brisk walk or run. Even such small measures have a beneficial effect, as do routine home activities such as running up the stairs, vacuum cleaning, mowing the lawn (as long as it is not with a 'sit-on' mower!), gardening and anything else that involves active physical movement and the expenditure of energy.

These simple activities provide a basis on which to build and a good place to start is simply to go for a walk as frequently as you can. Make sure that at least for some of the time, it is at an active, brisk pace with lengthened strides as this is best for achieving fitness. You may then wish to try longer and more challenging walks or move on to something else. A second extremely good form of exercise, that again can be carried out at very little cost, is swimming. This, like walking, is excellent for people of all ages.

Oriental forms of exercise

Oriental exercise techniques are particularly useful in anti-ageing for several reasons. They are suitable for people of all ages and can be continued into older age. They help to achieve flexibility of joints and muscles by a combination of stretching and relaxation, hence aiding the body to remain supple which is so very important during ageing. They exercise and relax both the body and the mind, in contrast to western forms of exercise which concentrate mainly upon physical training. The correct and regular practice of these techniques can have far-reaching beneficial effects, for example enhancing breathing and respiration, boosting the blood circulation and hence promoting the health of major organs, including the brain, heart, liver and kidneys. They are also excellent techniques for the control of stress – another important aspect of anti-ageing. Two oriental disciplines, yoga and T'ai-chi ch'uan are already quite well-known in the West but a third, Chi kung, is also excellent in anti-ageing.

Yoga

Yoga traces its origins to the ancient Indian civilisation of 4,000 years ago and, in its fullest development, is a complete way of life embracing all physical, mental, spiritual and emotional aspects of human existence. Awareness of breathing and ones inner, emotional and mental state is extremely important in yoga. The exercises are designed to encourage flexibility, promote correct breathing and enhance emotional and mental well-being, making use of periods of relaxation and meditation as part of the regime. There are many excellent books devoted to explaining yoga and exercises number into the thousands. A basic book on the subject can introduce you to the simpler yoga exercises, but a good way of learning is to join a class. Yoga is beneficial to all and some of the simpler exercises can be practised by people with physical disabilities and limitations. Alternative health practitioners may recommend yoga for the treatment of a number of disorders and its benefits have also been established in a number of orthodox medical trials.

T'ai-chi ch'uan

T'ai-chi ch'uan or simply T'ai chi is an ancient Chinese discipline developed by Taoist monks. Its aim is to achieve wholeness of mind, body and spirit through a series of exercises aimed at balancing the opposing life forces of Yin and Yang and the energy flow of

Qi. The exercises are best performed in the open air and are part of the daily routine for many thousands of Chinese people, from very young children to the elderly.

T'ai-chi requires patience, perseverance and a willingness to free the mind and emotions from everyday stresses and strains. It requires regular practice and it is best to learn from a qualified teacher by joining a class. It is a developmental form of exercise therapy with benefits that unfold gradually as time goes on. T'ai-chi is excellent for people of all ages, including the elderly and is beneficial in helping to maintain good posture, supple joints and muscles. It promotes restful sleep and the natural relief of stress. It enhances spiritual, emotional and mental wellbeing, helping to give the person a sense of calmness and peace and an ability to feel in control of his or her life – all attributes that are essential for positive ageing.

Chi kung

Chi kung or Qi gong is a series of exercises that, like T'ai-chi, is an ancient Chinese system practised by Taoists. The exercises are very gentle and are aimed at promoting correct breathing and meditation, making the person aware of his or her spiritual and emotional self. They are best performed in the open air and learnt from an experienced practitioner but can also be carried out on your own at home. Used regularly, Chi kung helps to control stress, promotes a healthy circulation and correct breathing, aids posture and suppleness and confers mental well-being and a sense of peace. Once again, these attributes are vital for those wishing to lead a long, healthy and active life and Chi kung is a safe and gentle exercise regime that is suitable for all age groups.

Other forms of relaxation and breathing exercise: simple techniques to use at home

Although the Oriental techniques described above are very useful, they may not be available to everyone. However, you can practise breathing, relaxation, simple exercises and meditation on your own at home in a manner that suits you best. As mentioned previously, there are very many books, magazine and newspaper articles featuring simple exercise routines that you may wish to use as a guide. But you can also devise simple techniques to suit yourself and these should be used in addition to the more vigorous forms of exercise referred to at the beginning of this section.

For example, relaxation exercises may take a variety of different forms but a commonly used method is termed progressive relaxation. In this, the person lies on his or her back on a comfortable surface such as a bed. Beginning with the head and face, groups of muscles are consciously contracted and 'held' for up to a minute before being relaxed. The process proceeds downwards through the neck, shoulders, chest, arms, abdomen, legs and feet until all the muscles are fully relaxed. A variation is to concentrate the mind on different areas of the body to induce them to relax completely. Breathing exercises are simply a matter of trying to become aware of the diaphragm and utilising it properly, instead of the chest and rib cage, in breathing. A good way to do this is to breathe in and out slowly and deeply through the nose, feeling the movement of the diaphragm and concentrating on filling and emptying the lungs properly. This can be practised at any time and you do not need to set aside a special time unless you particularly wish to do so. With regular practice, correct breathing will become normal for you, bringing the benefits of an improved circulation and oxygen supply to tissues and organs and relief from stress.

Simple exercises involve consciously utilising the full range of movements that are available to use. Examples include pulling the feet up towards you while sitting in a chair or rotating them at the ankles, raising the arms above the head and bending at the waist to reach towards the floor and keeping the back straight and holding on to a chair, slowly bending at the knees to a squatting position. As long as you are sensible and exercise with caution within the range of any physical limitations that you may have, you may well be surprised at the number of simple movements that are available to you.

Meditation

Meditation is the art of emptying the mind of all troublesome and intrusive thoughts in order to reach a state of complete relaxation and inner peace. In Eastern religion, it is used as a means of achieving a higher state of consciousness and spiritual enlightenment. Meditation confers many physical and mental benefits, lowering blood pressure, improving the circulation of the blood, relieving tension, stress and insomnia and promoting restful sleep. It can also help in the relief of pain and empowers people to cope more effectively with the stresses and strains of a busy, hectic life. All these factors have a part to play in anti-ageing and meditation can be regarded as a form of purely mental exercise, combined with correct breathing and relaxation.

Like all disciplines, meditation requires practice and perseverance but once the technique is mastered, many people find that they can slip into it quite easily, even amidst the hustle and bustle of everyday life. Some people prefer to meditate on their own from the start but others find it easier to join a group with a leader who can offer advice. If you wish to try and meditate on your own, choose a room or surroundings where you feel tranquil and peaceful and where you can be confident that you will not be interrupted. Sit on a comfortable chair or seat with your hands resting in your lap and close your eyes, if you wish. Concentrate on one calming, pleasant or neutral thought or look at a photograph, object or scene that has the same effect. Be aware of your breathing, ensuring that you can feel the movement of the diaphragm drawing air into and out of the lungs. Breathe deeply and slowly, filling and emptying the lungs completely, keeping your mouth shut so that air enters and leaves through the nose. Consciously relax all your muscles, beginning with the head and face, to ensure that there is no tension anywhere. If intrusive, exciting or troublesome thoughts intrude do not dwell on them but concentrate on the calm focus that you have chosen.

Continue in this way for the period of time that you have chosen and then allow yourself a few minutes to return to your usual state. It is a good idea to move your arms and legs around a little before standing up as you may feel light-headed. You may occasionally fall asleep during meditation but, in any event, you will feel mentally and physically refreshed and more ready to face the rest of the day's activities.

A Youthful Brain

THE HUMAN brain is a truly remarkable organ that not only tirelessly controls numerous functions of the body but also governs our individual character and emotions – the very essence that makes each person special and unique. The brain is constantly receiving and processing information from both within and without the body and sending out the appropriate responses and directions.

The brain is at its most potent during early childhood when neural pathways are being established and an immense amount of information is received, recorded and stored. In early adult life, there is a net daily loss of brain cells and these are not replaced. However, this occurs in a controlled manner and is compensated for, to a certain extent, by the remaining cells so that there is usually very little noticeable decline in capability until much later in life.

Memory

The area that is most usually affected and where loss of capability may be noticed is in the workings of memory. Usually the decline is slight until advanced old age when memory problems become much more common. In elderly people, there is a build up of plaques of abnormal, dysfunctional material and this is especially abundant in the brain of those suffering from Alzheimer's disease. The plaques are believed to occur as a result of increasing free radical damage and as a natural consequence of ageing. However, their exact relationship with the development of dementia is still unclear as the brains of all elderly people show changes but not all suffer from Alzheimer's disease.

Decision making and problem solving

The ability to make decisions and solve problems may be affected but usually, people just require a little more time to reach a solution. The wisdom and experience of older age often more than compensates for the hasty decision making of youth. The good news is that there are several ways in which we can endeavour to protect our brain from natural, age-related damage and these fall naturally into two groups. The first group includes diet and the use of helpful supplements to support the brain and the second involves mental exercise – keeping the brain sharp through constant stimulation and intellectual challenge.

Brain food

A good diet for the brain basically involves following

the nutritional guidelines discussed in the preceding section. Oily fish and vegetable oils are good for the brain as are plenty of antioxidant-rich fruits and vegetables. Eat plenty of foods containing selenium, carotenoids, vitamin C, vitamin E, the B vitamins and coenzyme Q10 or use supplements, if necessary.

One non-food supplement that has been found to be particularly helpful in boosting the brain is an extract prepared from the Maidenhair tree, Ginkgo biloba. This improves blood circulation, particularly in the smallest blood vessels, the capillaries, across which the exchange of gases and nutrients takes place. Taking Ginkgo biloba improves the blood, oxygen and nutrient supply to the brain but the compound has other properties as well. It is a potent antioxidant but it also has a powerful effect upon intellectual faculties, especially improving memory, concentration and the ability to carry out mental tasks. It has a protective effect upon nerve cells and has anti-inflammatory properties that are particularly useful in the relief of asthma. Scientific studies have shown that Ginkgo biloba can help to improve the memory and mental performance of people suffering from early to moderate Alzheimer's dementia and slow up the progression of the disease.

Ginkgo biloba is taken by many thousands of people throughout the world and although it has excellent properties, it can rarely produce side effects. These include rash, headache, lightheadedness and bleeding irregularities in women. It is available in capsule form from chemist shops and pharmacies and usually needs to be taken for about two months before its effects become noticeable.

Brain exercises

Mental exercises for the brain can take as many different forms as physical exercises for the body. If you find the whole idea a little off-putting, do not worry! You are already performing many mental exercises, just as a result of everyday living. The idea here is to merely stretch and challenge the brain just a little bit more so that it will remain alert and perform even better. So, first of all, how can you challenge your brain as you go about your daily routine? The possibilities are almost endless and you will almost certainly be able to come up with a few ideas of our own but here are just a few examples to get you started.

Even if your work is mentally and physically exhausting and you feel like doing nothing except slumping in front of the television set every evening, try to make the effort to do something different that will utilise the brain. You could, for example, read a quality newspaper, magazine or interesting book and think about what you have read and perhaps share your thoughts with someone else. You could attempt to do the crossword/puzzle page, write that letter that you have been meaning to write, play a game of chess or spend some time devising a plan for a DIY project or relating to a favourite sport or hobby. If you are prepared to offer your services to any voluntary or community-based group, you will almost certainly find yourself utilising your organisational and planning skills and hence exercising your brain in a very positive way. You may think that these things are too trivial and simple to make any difference, but just as the fitness of the body can be boosted in simple ways, so can the fitness of the mind. The important thing with both physical and mental exercise is not to allow yourself to be lazy! If you keep challenging your brain by following up new ideas, interests and skills, you will help it to remain active and alert throughout life.

As mentioned above, the most common noticeable area in which ageing affects the brain is in the workings of the memory. However, the memory can be sharpened and improved by the performance of simple exercises and it is important to take the time and trouble to carry these out as we age, in order to maintain our memory in good working order. Once again, with a little thought and effort you can consciously exercise your memory as you go about your daily life. For example, instead of looking at your shopping list when you go to the supermarket, try to remember what is on it and check at the end to see how many items you have missed. When you pass someone in the street, quickly try to memorise as many details about that person as you can manage, as though you were later going to have to give a description to the police. Or, you could think about an outing or event that you attended during the previous week.

Try to remember every single detail about what happened – timing, how you got there, the clothes that you wore, the food that you ate, the people that you went with, met or talked to and the topics of conversation. If you went to a play, film or concert – recall as many details as you can manage. When you are reading something, memorise a few lines and then make an effort to recall them a few hours later or on the following day. These are just a few examples and you will probably be able to come up with several more for yourself.

Also, there are the more familiar memory tests such as looking at a group or list of objects for ten seconds and then shutting your eyes and seeing how many of them you can recall. If you try this regularly, you will soon be able to remember more items, especially if you employ a technique known as 'chunking'. This involves mentally organising the items into similar groups, if possible, which is more effective than simply trying to remember things at random.

There are several old-fashioned games that test the memory. For example, the one where, for each letter of the alphabet, every person in the group in turn has to name a country, river, animal, flower, etc. beginning with that letter. Hence memory exercises do not have to be dull, nor should they be regarded with trepidation as something that you might fail. It is best to look upon them as a bit of fun, with the additional benefit of developing the memory and keeping it in trim. A high proportion of our daily thought processes rely on the use of memory, from reflecting on the day's events to recalling past experiences to help solve a present problem. With a little thought and effort, we can all find ways of exercising our memory more effectively and there are also many helpful books available on this subject.

Keeping the brain and memory exercised has other benefits that are not immediately apparent. Research has shown that mental exercise regulates the balance of natural chemicals released by the brain that help it to work efficiently. Mental exercise confers a sense of well-being and satisfaction and boosts self-confidence. We feel pleased when we have managed to grasp and understand a difficult intellectual concept or, through our own logical thought processes, have solved some challenging problem. The intellectual problems and challenges may vary from person to person but we all have the ability to exercise our minds and can reap the benefits of doing so.

Regular mental exercise appears to boost the immune system and aids the ability to cope with stress. People who carry this out are less likely to suffer from depression and usually maintain a positive outlook on life. Feeling self-confident and positive are both aspects of anti-ageing, allowing people to look forward to the future and welcome what lies ahead. As we shall see below, devising a plan for positive thinking and adhering to it, is one of the best anti-ageing strategies that you can employ.

Finally, do not forget that like the rest of the body, the brain benefits from physical exercise too, through increased blood flow and oxygen supply and the sights, sounds and stimulation provided by the use of muscles. Your brain may feel exhausted after a long day in the office but if you can fit in an evening walk or other form of exercise that you enjoy, you will be surprised at how re-energised it will make you feel.

Mind and Spirit

S O FAR, we have considered the intellect and memory and seen the importance of keeping these challenged and exercised in order to maintain a youthful brain. But there is, of course, another unique aspect to every human being, governed by the brain, that is our spiritual, contemplative side – or soul, in religious terms. The spirit is a difficult thing to pin down. It involves the intellect and emotions and the unique 'essence' that makes each one of us who we are – a person who is different from everyone else. It finds a natural home in the acceptance and practice of religion, but even those without any religious beliefs are usually prepared to acknowledge the existence of the spirit.

Anti-ageing and the spiritual self

Surveys consistently show that those who follow and practise a religion, which almost invariably involves having faith in something unseen and greater than themselves, fare better in certain aspects of anti-ageing. They experience less anxiety, stress and depression and although they may not live any longer than those who are non-religious, they often have an inner serenity and certainty that banishes any fear of ageing and death. Religious faith often confers a sense of self-worth and value through service to others and a belief that the person's life is taken care of, both before and after death. Of course, this is not to say that those who are not religious cannot find this sense of serenity – many do – but those with a religious faith seem to have a head start!

You may or may not have any religious faith. Since this is a matter of belief in something more profound than everyday human experience, religion is not something that can be just lightly accepted or discarded. However, it is a good idea to remain open to the ideas and beliefs of the various religious faiths and to be sufficiently interested to discuss them with others. You will at least understand the religious beliefs of others and at some stage in life, you may find that you are more receptive to these ideas and wish to examine them again.

There are ways other than those of formal religion to explore and satisfy the spiritual nature that every human being possesses. A little self-examination may be needed to discover how this can be achieved. It may be through contemplation of art, literature or nature – going into the countryside or another wild place, watching the motion of the sea, gardening or, very often, spending time and effort on some worthwhile project and helping other people. (The practice of Eastern forms of exercise, and meditation, described above, are other helpful ways of putting people in touch with their spiritual selves).

Every person should take time to do what feels right for themselves. This makes sound sense from the point of view of anti-ageing, producing a vital sense of fulfilment, feeling at ease with oneself and having a direction and purpose to follow. Neglect in this area may cause the opposite: dissatisfaction and restlessness. These are negative feelings that can contribute to other problems such as stress and the development of mild depression, both of which are unhelpful for successful anti-ageing.

Devising a plan for positive thinking

Numerous studies have proved, beyond any shadow of doubt, the power of the mind in influencing the state of the body. Those who are able to maintain a positive outlook and who remain determined, even in the face of adversity, fare better than those who are passive and accepting. For example, surveys of people being treated for cancer have consistently shown that those who are determined to fight the disease in whatever way they can, survive for longer and have a better quality of life, than those who do not.

It is thought that positive thinking affects the subtle, biochemical functions of the brain, promoting the release of helpful substances that boost the immune system and the health of the body. It is, of course, easier to practise positive thinking if you are currently in good health and have no pressing, outstanding worries or concerns. If you are ill or presently feeling overwhelmed by worries in life, it is possibly insensitive to exhort you to think positively as this may be beyond your present resources. However, there are techniques and strategies in this book that may help you (e.g. exercise, how to recognize and manage stress and alternative therapies) and finding out more about these is, in itself, a step on the road towards adopting a more positive frame of mind.

If you take a few moments to analyse it, you will see that devising and following a plan of positive thinking is largely concerned with anti-ageing! Think for a few moments about the things that, deep down, worry and concern you and write them down. You will see that most of them concern events that you fear may happen in the future, either imminently or at a much later date. On most peoples' list are fears concerning old age, disease and disability, either affecting themselves or those dear to them. The first step to thinking more positively is to realize that many of these things MAY NOT HAPPEN and, in any event, they belong to the future and are not happening now. To counteract them and the negative impact that they are likely to be having on your life at a subconscious level, write down, read and repeat as many positive statements about yourself as you can think of. You

will, no doubt, be able to come up with many of
your own but here are a few ideas to get you started!

When you look in the mirror as you are getting
up, say:

Today I am as young as I shall ever be.
I intend to enjoy myself and all the events that
    the day will bring.
I will cope well with all the day's activities, in-
    cluding ...
I am glad to be XX years old.
I enjoy life, especially ...... and have many things
    to look forward to.
I am pleased with all the knowledge I have gained
    and shall continue to learn many new things
    in the future.
I cannot change the past but I *can* make choices
    for the future.
I believe in myself and my ability to make changes
    that will make my life even better.
I intend to do all that I can to look after myself
    and to remain healthy and fit.

Try to bring yourself to make some of these
affirmations out loud, even if you feel self-conscious
about it at first. If this makes you smile or laugh, so much
the better – laughter is good for you (*see* below). Think
about your list of affirmations when you have a spare
moment during the day and repeat them if you can or

else jot them down. Doing this really does have a beneficial effect in helping you to feel good about yourself and in remaining positive about the future.

Expand the ideas outlined above and imagine yourself in ten years time, concentrating on all the better aspects that you can think of. Perhaps you will be retired and at last will have time to do the things that you enjoy, have children who will finally be independent, will have paid off your mortgage or become more financially secure. Perhaps you will have become a grandparent or maybe you can imagine yourself carrying out some pet project or even embarking upon an entirely new kind of life somewhere else. You will still feel fit, active and healthy and fully able to enjoy your life. Indulge in occasional daydreaming about this life that lies ahead of you and this will help you to keep looking forward to the future. The life that you are imagining may not come to pass but it has a better chance of doing so if you think in this way and do not allow any negative thoughts to creep in.

Laughter is good for the mind and the body and causes certain physiological changes that enhance wellbeing. A surprising number of muscles are used during a bout of laughter and there is also a release of arousal hormones from the adrenal glands. Breathing rate is increased so that more oxygen is made available and the heart and circulation are stimulated. Following a period of hearty laughter, the muscles are totally relaxed and we may even feel weak for a little while. There is a release of all muscle tension and a complete absence of any sense of stress. In a social setting, laughter shared with others promotes bonding and friendship and lowers any sense of stress, tension or rivalry. During laughter, subtle physiological changes take place in the brain and there is a lessening of the perception of pain. Laughter also seems to boost the immune system and lower blood pressure. Research has shown that those who laugh a lot generally suffer from fewer illnesses and this may be because these people have a happy and optimistic outlook on life.

You may feel that there is not a great deal for you to laugh at and that laughter does not come naturally to you. But making the effort to smile is a first step and is one of the most positive things that you can do in your dealings with other people. Smiling confers some of the benefits of laughter and is a step on the way towards being able to laugh outright. Try to find something to laugh at each day; read an amusing article or book, or watch or listen to a comedy programme. Remember an incident that you found hilarious and let the memory of it cause you to smile and laugh just now. Better still, share it with someone else so that they can benefit too.

Positive thinking and laughter are anti-ageing strategies for both mind and body and also help to counteract the effects of periods of stress, which are a universal part of human existence. Stress plays a major role in life and contributes to many known ageing effects and to the development of illness. It is worth examining it in a little more detail so that we can learn to recognize and understand stress and control its negative effects.

How to recognize and manage stress

Stress can be defined as a state of physical and mental tension caused by certain external or internal factors in a person's life. The causes of stress are varied and numerous, as are people's responses to them. The cause may be something obvious, that would produce symptoms of stress in almost anyone, such as extreme physical danger with the expectation of imminent death or disaster. Or it may be a far more subtle, mental anxiety sufficient to cause extreme stress in one individual but a matter of indifference in another.

Stress is part of the human condition, needed to maintain alertness for life and hence, to some extent, it is unavoidable. All mammals have evolved similar physiological adaptations to deal with external, physical stresses. These adaptations involve the release of hormones from the adrenal glands and certain nerve endings and which prepare the body for 'fright, flight or fight'. The body and mind are rendered tense and alert, ready for immediate action and certain processes, such as digestion and excretion, which are not required for this are temporarily suspended.

This is obviously appropriate in circumstances of

physical danger but people react in the same way to emotional and psychological stress as well. In these instances, the physiological reactions are not needed and are therefore unhelpful and they can cause harm, especially if prolonged. Examples of emotional and psychological stress include being on the receiving end of verbal bullying, unpleasant or difficult relationships, illness or suffering of a loved one and the continual pressure posed by too great a workload. Many people experience both short and long-term stress of this sort and it produces both physical and mental symptoms, some of which are more obvious than others, so that a person is not necessarily aware that he or she is suffering from the effects of stress. This is due to the fact that the mind and body adapt, to a certain extent, to the stressed state so that signs and symptoms go unrecognized.

Symptoms that frequently occur include: feelings of panic; shortness of breath or breathing difficulties; palpitations; loss of appetite or comfort eating; anxiety; insomnia; irritability; impatience; angry outbursts; unexplained pains, especially digestive and/or abdominal; muscle tension; frequent headaches; tiredness, inability to concentrate, forgetfulness, indecision; and increased reliance on alcohol, smoking, coffee, etc.

Prolonged stress is a serious condition that is known to increase the risk of developing certain illnesses, some of which are life threatening or shorten life expectancy. These include high blood pressure, heart attack, angina, circulatory disorders, migraine, ulcers, mental breakdown, depression, irritable bowel syndrome and suppression of the immune system leading to increased susceptibility to infection.

The causes of stress may or may not be obvious to the individual concerned and so the first step, if you are experiencing symptoms, is to conduct a detailed and honest assessment of your life. In particular, try to pinpoint the times when you feel most stressed in order to identify exact causes. Once the causes are known, it is necessary to deal with these problems, beginning with those that are most significant, whether they relate to home, family life, other relationships or financial matters.

Initially, many people feel that dealing with their problems, the causes of their stress, is impossible. However, taking charge of the problems by bringing them out into the open and discussing them frankly with work colleagues, family and friends are vital steps in managing stress. Often, people feel inhibited about discussing their problems because they believe that they should be capable of coping on their own and they feel inadequate. Another common mistake is for the sufferer to believe that he is the only one experiencing problems while all around him seem to be fine. However, once problems are aired, a person is usually surprised to discover that many others have shared similar experiences. Usually, this brings a great sense of relief and an immediate lessening of stress. If you feel reluctant to discuss the causes of your stress with others, try to overcome your inhibitions and talk to one person whom you trust. Realizing the harm that the stress is causing you and that it may even be taking years off your life, will hopefully provide the necessary incentive. If you prefer to do so, talk to your family doctor.

Once the process of identifying and dealing with the causes of stress is initiated, there are other measures that can help. Firstly, it is essential to make time for recreational and social activities that will help you to relax, give you something to look forward to and divert your attention away from your problems. All these are stress-busting measures. It is equally essential to take plenty of exercise as this encourages restful sleep which is, in itself, an important part of stress management. Take up one of the Eastern exercise disciplines described previously and practise breathing and relaxation, meditation and positive thinking. Some alternative therapies such as herbal remedies, homeopathy, aromatherapy, massage and visualisation therapy are also very helpful in the relief of stress. A good anti-ageing diet is vital at all times but especially important for those who are stressed.

As we have seen, adrenal gland hormones which prepare the body for 'fright, flight or fight' are heavily involved in the body's reaction to stress. However, the adrenal glands produce other hormones which regulate the electrolytes (salts) and water balance in the body and are involved in energy metabolism. Prolonged stress can adversely affect these important functions and lead to depletion of the body's vital potassium stores. Hence it is a good idea to ensure that you are eating plenty of potassium-rich foods and obtaining plenty of vitamins through eating a good and varied diet.

Strengthening the
Immune System

AS HAS been seen from the discussion in the previous section, *Theories about ageing*, the immune system is the protective shield that not only keeps us well but also, it is believed, eventually plays a part in causing us to age. Hence supporting the immune system in as many ways as we can is one of the most important anti-ageing strategies that we can employ.

The immune system can be helped in several ways, some of which can be roughly grouped under the now familiar headings of diet, nutrition and lifestyle choices (including exercise, stress management and positive thinking). Other methods include the judicial use of non-food supplements and drugs, which in the case of some products is controversial, and also the approaches advocated by some alternative therapies.

To safeguard the immune system, you should ensure that you are eating a good, anti-ageing diet containing plenty of natural antioxidants. Eating a wide variety of foods, including plenty of fruit and vegetables, unrefined carbohydrates, fish, chicken and lean meat will ensure that you receive a good intake of the vitamins and minerals that are essential for the correct functioning of the immune system. Animal fats, sugar, refined carbohydrates, alcohol and coffee should be consumed sparingly. Foods rich in vitamin C and zinc are particularly important. Zinc deficiency is a common cause of lowered immunity especially among the elderly who may benefit from taking a multi-vitamin and mineral supplement.

Regular exercise seems to benefit the immune system, perhaps through the boost that it gives to the heart and circulation. As we have seen, positive thinking influences bodily health and, in the event of illness, appears sometimes to be able to help the immune system fight off the effects of disease. One of the best ways to support the immune system is simply to be careful about the way we lead our life. Long, stress-filled days, late nights, lack of sleep, irregular mealtimes, smoking and excess consumption of alcohol are all factors that are likely to result in lowered immunity and the onset of illness and exhaustion, as many people discover to their cost. We may be able to do very little about all the unseen, external pollutants and environmental factors that assail the immune system every day. But each of us can and should choose a lifestyle that is supportive of our body's natural defences if we wish to lead a long and healthy life. One further point, and one that is frequently overlooked, is the importance of avoiding infection, especially in older age when any illness is potentially more damaging. It is sensible not to seek the close company of anyone who is suffering from a cold or other viral infection, and also to try and avoid passing on any such illness yourself.

Several supplements are available that are held to be particularly helpful for the immune system. Some of these are more tried and tested than others while a few are controversial. Almost all are natural products, either found in foods or occurring naturally within the body, or else herbal extracts derived from plants. In the list below, only those that are not described elsewhere are discussed in detail.

As mentioned above, vitamin C and zinc are helpful and can be safely taken at recommended doses in supplement form. Although some doctors and health experts remain unconvinced, many people who take large doses of vitamin C are convinced that it helps them to stay free of everyday infections such as the common cold.

Among the herbal remedies, extracts from the aloe vera plant are beneficial to the immune system. Aloe vera is used externally for the healing of minor skin conditions but it also appears to have anti-inflammatory properties when taken by mouth. It is believed to stimulate immune system cells called macrophages, that engulf foreign particles, acting as free-ranging scavengers. Aloe vera is also particularly helpful in the treatment of allergies and possibly some other conditions as well.

An extract derived from the olive tree is believed to boost the immune system to fight off ubiquitous infections such as thrush, the common cold and influenza. Extract of Cat's Claw (a South American rainforest plant) is also held to have anti-infective and anti-inflammatory properties.

Green tea is a potent antioxidant and is believed to have anti-cancer properties and to act as a general immune system booster. It is also available in supplement form for those who do not enjoy drinking the tea.

There are many other herbal, homeopathic and naturopathic remedies that may be recommended by therapists to boost the immune system. It is best to consult a practitioner and/or read one of the many books that are available if you wish to find out more about these.

Several substances, which occur naturally in the body but which generally decline with age, have been found to act as boosters for the immune system. Carnosine and co-enzyme Q_{10} are found in certain foods but can also be taken as supplements and are believed, by anti-ageing experts, to be particularly useful. Another natural substance that cannot, however, be found in sufficient quantities in food, is an amino acid (protein) called dimethylglycine (DMG). This is believed by some experts to boost several elements of the immune system in their task of disease and infection prevention. It can be safely taken as a supplement and has many enthusiastic supporters but many medical experts believe that there is no evidence to support the claims made for its beneficial effects.

Some of the most controversial, non-food supplements which may have to be administered by injection, are naturally occurring hormones. These are said to have multiple anti-ageing effects, of which boosting the immune system is one important function. They include growth hormone, (somatotrophin), dehydroepiandrosterone (DHE) and melatonin. These are discussed in more detail below.

Finally, several alternative therapies are beneficial and supportive of the immune system including Ayurvedic medicine, flotation therapy, herbal medicine, homeopathy, hydrotherapy, naturopathy, laughter therapy, light therapy and visualization. These are briefly described in a later section.

Conventional Medicine

ALTHOUGH we are perhaps not accustomed to associating conventional medicine and surgery with anti-ageing, a few moments' consideration enables us to see that a great deal of modern medical practice is concerned with just that. This has become particularly true in recent years, with the growing interest in preventative medicine as opposed to the treatment of disease alone. Screening and genetic testing so that preventative action can be taken if the results indicate the likelihood of disease can be considered in this light, as can the advice that is now routinely available from doctors' surgeries on a wide range of health and lifestyle aspects.

Any medical or surgical treatment that corrects an age-related disease or condition can be considered to be anti-ageing. The most successful examples are those that restore mobility, vigour or vitality which have been reduced or lost and which have a rejuvenating effect upon the whole person. The restoration of better health obviously restores a higher quality of life and helps the person to achieve a more positive state of mind. These, as we have seen, are themselves important aspects of anti-ageing. In many instances and certainly in individual cases, these procedures save and extend life and may make it possible for the people concerned to achieve their full life span.

Familiar examples include hip and knee replacements, coronary by-pass surgery, cataract removal, and hormone replacement therapy for menopausal women. Hormone replacement therapy or HRT has proved to be a particularly useful treatment for many women, not only removing unpleasant menopausal symptoms but also slowing down the accelerated rate of bone loss that is a natural consequence of declining oestrogen levels (*see* Menopause and osteoporosis in section Selected examples of age-related conditions and their treatment, page 192).

Taking HRT for five or even ten years significantly reduces the risk of fractures in elderly women. Fractures in old age, especially of major bones and weight-bearing joints, are particularly serious as they often do not heal properly. Complications and trauma from these injuries can be a cause of death and for this reason many conventional doctors advocate HRT for their older female patients. The success of this therapy may be one of the factors that initially encouraged interest in the use of other hormonal treatments for anti-ageing.

Although controversial, scientific research using

early human embryonic stem cells offers future hope to many people with diseased tissues and organs, including those suffering from age-related damage. The cells are obtained from very early stage human embryos and are then cultured in the laboratory. They are called stem cells because at this stage, they are not differentiated and have the potential to form different kinds of tissue, depending upon the environment in which they are placed. Treating them with various drugs and chemicals encourages them to develop into particular cell types. Scientific researchers are excited about the prospect of being able to transplant appropriately treated stem cells into damaged tissues and organs in order to effect repairs. In August 2001, Israeli scientists announced an exciting breakthrough in embryonic stem cell research, having succeeded in growing cardiomyocytes – immature heart cells. Although the research is still in its early stages, the scientists are convinced that these cells would become fully functioning heart cells, if transplanted. This exciting development offers the hope that in the future, many people with heart disease will be helped by the introduction of cells that can take over the functions of the damaged areas.

Many other areas of scientific and medical research – into the causes and treatment of cancer, Alzheimer's disease, arthritis, heart and circulatory disease and autoimmune disorders, for example – continue to produce promising breakthroughs for the future. Many are expected to get to the stage of clinical trials and hence treatment regimes within the next five, ten or fifteen years. Hence developments in both mainstream and specialist anti-ageing medicine offer hopeful prospects for all who are ageing in the 21st century which, of course, includes us all!

Hormonal anti-ageing treatments

As discussed in an earlier section (*see* Why Do We Age?, page 17), many experts believe that the natural decline in the level of various hormones that occurs as we grow older is responsible, to a great extent, for ageing and its effects. Not surprisingly, these experts believe that the key to slowing down ageing is to replenish one or more of these lost hormones and to restore them to the levels at which they existed in youth.

Human growth hormone

Human growth hormone is considered by many anti-ageing specialists to be one of the key factors involved in ageing. In order to understand why this may be so, it is necessary to look at this hormone in a little more detail.

HGH is a large, complex peptide (protein) molecule that is produced and secreted by the anterior lobe of the pituitary gland at the base of the brain. Also known as somatotrophin, this important hormone controls protein synthesis, i.e. growth in children, and is necessary for vital tissue repair, healing and replacement of cells throughout adult life. Not surprisingly, HGH is produced at high levels during childhood but the amount has plummeted by the age of 20 and then continues to decline steadily through each succeeding decade of life. By the age of 60, the level of HGH has fallen to a fraction of what it was in childhood. The appearance of the physical effects of ageing directly corresponds with the decline in human growth hormone.

From the late 1950s, HGH extracted from pituitary glands after death was used to treat children suffering from a lack of the hormone in order to induce them to grow normally and to avoid dwarfism. In the 1980s, a synthetic form of HGH was produced and in the 1990s, clinical trials in elderly adults were carried out for the first time. In almost all cases, the results were reported to be dramatic, reversing the effects of ageing by about 20 years.

In the early trials, some significant side effects occurred including enlargement of breasts, in both males and females, carpal tunnel syndrome (painful wrists), fluid retention, increased risk of diabetes, joint pains, headaches and high blood pressure. However, reducing the dose of HGH appeared to produce the desired anti-ageing results without adverse side effects. Specifically, treatment with HGH appears to reduce body fat (particularly abdominal), increases the thickness and elasticity of the skin and reduces wrinkles, strengthens bones, increases muscle mass, significantly improves immune system function with greater resilience to infection and faster healing of wounds. Sexual function, intellectual capabilities including memory and feeling more positive about life are also said to improve and energy levels increase. In addition, patients suffering from AIDS, Parkinson's disease and Alzheimer's dementia have all been reported to show improvement after HGH treatment.

Normally, HGH is secreted by the pituitary gland in response to controlling chemicals released from the hypothalamus in the brain. Once it enters the bloodstream, HGH remains there for only a few minutes, being taken up by the liver and converted into various other peptide molecules, particularly insulin-like growth factor-one or IGF-1. IGF-1 then mediates many of the physiological effects of HGH. HGH itself is naturally secreted in short bursts during the early phases of sleep but its secretion is boosted by hard exercise, adrenaline release during emotional stress and in periods of calorie-restricted eating. Interestingly, studies in laboratory animals have shown that their longevity is significantly increased by a lifetime of slight under-eating. It can be postulated that this may be partly due to an increased availability of growth hormone in these animals.

HGH and IGF-1 affect the physiological and

biochemical functions of almost all body cells in highly complex ways. Replacement therapy with HGH appears to literally turn the clock back, producing tissues and organs that are biologically younger than the chronological age of the body they inhabit. Supplementation has to be given by injection on a daily basis and must be under the supervision of a suitably qualified physician at an anti-ageing clinic. The blood levels of IGF-1 (which remains in the circulation) are monitored with the aim of ultimately producing a level of hormone consistent with that of a person aged about 25 years. The dosage of hormone must be tailored to the individual person and the cost of the treatment is high. It is also far from 'mainstream' and is available at very few centres within the UK, although this may change in the future.

Secretagogues

Secretagogues are substances that, it is claimed, stimulate the body's natural production of growth hormone by the pituitary gland. Most secretagogues are naturally occurring organic compounds such as certain amino acids which are found within the body. Others are plant extracts that are said to stimulate HGH production. Most of these products are the subject of intense scientific scrutiny and if the claims made about any of them are substantiated, they are likely to become very important in the field of anti-ageing.

Gamma Hydroxy Butyric acid

Gamma Hydroxy Butyric acid or GHB is one of the secretagogues for which significant claims have been made with regard to its effect on levels of growth hormone. Although a natural form of the chemical exists in the body, synthetic GHB is an anaesthetic drug and in several studies, it has been shown to promote the stages of sleep in which growth hormone is released. This resulted in elevated amounts of HGH and IGF-1 (human growth hormone) being detected in the blood, without causing any change in insulin or blood sugar. The latter result is encouraging because injections of HGH itself do affect the insulin/glucose balance and increase the risk of the development of diabetes.

Further studies have been carried out with an almost identical chemical, gamma butyrolactone or GBL, that was given by mouth as a dietary supplement. This was taken in a lesser amount that did not induce sleep and was also found to promote HGH release without affecting insulin/blood sugar levels.

However, while some researchers believe that it is safe to take GHB or GBL as a growth hormone promoter, many others have very grave concerns. Serious adverse consequences have been reported in some patients who were taking GHB alongside other potent drugs and alcohol. Those who support the use of GHB and GBL maintain that its detractors have not studied the evidence properly and seem determined to prevent the widespread availability of a useful anti-ageing product. At the present time, GHB and GBL can be obtained in Europe but have been banned in some states in the USA.

Dehydroepiadrosterone

Dehydroepiadrosterone or DHEA or is a naturally occurring androgen (male steroid hormone) produced by the adrenal glands which are located near the kidneys. It is also secreted in smaller amounts by the testicles and ovaries. The level of DHEA reaches a high point at around the age of 25 years and then progressively and steadily declines. It has been discovered that those in better health in older age generally have higher blood levels of DHEA.

Supplementation with DHEA has been found, in some trials, to be helpful in the treatment of ageing. It appears to boost bone density in postmenopausal women and encourage loss of fat and increased muscle bulk in people of both sexes. Extra DHEA is said to be able to help improve mood and counteract depression in the elderly and to boost memory function. It may boost libido and help with other male sexual performance problems. It is believed to be valuable in the treatment, and possibly the prevention, of a range of autoimmune diseases, that may, in themselves, be age-related. Their number include systemic lupus erythematosus, multiple sclerosis, rheumatoid arthritis and ulcerative colitis. AIDS patients have also noticed improvement following DHEA treatment.

Most DHEA supplements are in the form of capsules or tablets but it is sometimes administered as drops under the tongue or in chewing gum. It is manufactured in the laboratory from a precursor (diosgenin) found in Mexican wild yams.

Even those who support the use of DHEA accept that it should be taken with caution, especially by women. No one aged under 40 years should take DHEA and high doses must be avoided as there may be toxic, damaging effects on the liver. DHEA is also a precursor of oestrogen. It should not be used by pregnant or nursing mothers or any person, male or female, who is either suffering or at risk from a hormone-dependent cancer, i.e. of the womb, breasts, ovaries, testicles or prostate gland.

Many other clinicians and researchers have expressed grave concerns about the use of DHEA, believing that any short term health gains are offset by the potential for serious side effects and increased risk of liver damage and reproductive cancers.

Melatonin
Melatonin came to fame a few years ago and was briefly hailed as an anti-ageing 'wonder drug'. Data proving the claims that have been made for it is scanty but it remains a popular and apparently safe anti-ageing remedy with many people swearing by its beneficial effects.

Melatonin is secreted by the pineal gland, which is a small mass of specialised nerve tissue located near the centre of the brain. Melatonin is involved in the regulation of circadian rhythms in mammals, i.e. the changes in activity, behaviour and physiology that occur over a 24-hour period such as the determination of periods of sleep and wakefulness. In humans, as in other mammals, it regulates the body's internal, 24-hour clock and melatonin release is high during the hours of darkness but low and suppressed by daylight.

The one claim that can be made for melatonin – and one that makes sense – is that it can help people with jet lag, particularly those such as airline crews who regularly cross time zones. The other benefits that have been laid at its door are more difficult to substantiate but include relief of depression, particularly Seasonal Affective Disorder (SAD) since this is more prevalent during the dark winter months, when natural melatonin levels could be expected to be high, it is difficult to see how supplementation helps.

Melatonin is said to have potent antioxidant properties and may help to counteract ageing effects; it may be of benefit to those suffering from Alzheimer's dementia; it has been claimed to have protective properties against certain cancers, i.e. of the breast and prostate gland; and it may be beneficial in the treatment of multiple sclerosis, heart disease and epilepsy.

Melatonin is believed to be safe and no adverse side effects have been reported but there is no recommended dose. Dosages vary from between 0.3mg to 6mg for the treatment of jet lag and sleep disorders. Since this is a hormonal treatment, it is not recommended for anyone suffering from cancer, immune system disorder, including autoimmune diseases, or women trying to conceive or who are pregnant.

Pregnenolone
Pregnenolone is a naturally occurring hormone-like substance that is produced within the body from cholesterol. It acts as a basic precursor for all the human steroid hormones, e.g. male and female sex hormones and all the adrenal gland hormones. These include the glucocorticosteroids (cortisol and cortisone) which regulate glucose metabolism and are responsible for stress responses. It is believed that one of the main anti-ageing benefits of pregnenolone is in stress reduction. As with so many hormones, pregnenolone levels fall with increasing age. Some researchers believe that in youth, pregnenolone acts as a general anti-stress chemical as well as a precursor necessary for the manufacture of steroid hormones. As levels fall with ageing, its anti-stress capability may be removed because there is not enough present for it to fulfil both its roles within the body. Supplementation with pregnenolone appears to be safe and it is alleged that by lowering stress, it also boosts other intellectual functions, particularly improving memory.

It is said to have anti-depressant, mood-enhancing effects.

Other beneficial effects have been reported, particularly anti-inflammatory and anti-allergic properties which have helped some sufferers from arthritis. Pregnenolone was used quite extensively in the 1940s and interest in it has recently revived in the field of anti-ageing.

Non-food anti-ageing supplements
Gerovital

Gerovital or GH_3, KH_3 is one of the original anti-ageing drugs that first came to fame in the 1950s and 1960s, when it attracted a following that included film stars and politicians. Gerovital was invented by a Romanian specialist who designated it GH_3, a combination of the dental anaesthetic procaine, with small quantities of potassium, metabisulphate, disodium phosphate and benzoic acid. These added ingredients act as buffers and stabilisers and delay the breaking down of the procaine into its two constituent parts, DEAE (diethylaminoethanol) and PABA (para-aminobenzoic acid). DEAE and PABA are both useful chemicals that naturally occur in the body. DEAE promotes the production of neurotransmitters, such as acetylcholine, which are essential for the passage of electrical impulses and hence for the correct functioning of the nervous system. PABA stimulates the bacterial flora of the hind gut to produce vitamin K. However, GH3 appears to have a special property which is to be able to weakly and reversibly reduce the level of the brain enzyme MAO (monamine oxidase). Monamine oxidase is an essential enzyme that removes excess levels of brain neurochemicals (neurohormones and neurotransmitters) particularly dopamine, serotonin and noradrenaline (norepinephrine).

From middle age onwards, levels of MAO start to rise while that of the brain neurochemicals declines. A consequence of this is that there is a decline in memory, ability to concentrate and notably an increased incidence of depression. By acting as a reversible MAO inhibitor – an MAOI – GH3 is claimed to have a directly beneficial effect, improving memory and concentration, relieving depression and insomnia, and also improving muscle strength, activity and energy levels. Other specific anti-ageing claims are also made for GH3 and another very similar preparation, which is half as strong, called KH3. It is said to rejuvenate cells, particularly muscle cells, strengthen the skin and remove wrinkles, relieve stress and be beneficial in the treatment of a wide range of age-related conditions. Relief of stress and counteracting the life-long effects of cortisol (the stress hormone), particularly by protecting an area of the brain known as the hippocampus, is believed by the supporters of GH3, to be probably its most important, hitherto unsuspected role in anti-ageing.

Side effects are reported to be few but GH3/KH3 should not be used by those taking prescribed anti-depressants or who have a known allergy to procaine. As with any supplements, GH3 is best taken under medical advice. It must be said that although many people have found GH3 to be helpful, the majority of the medical profession do not accept that the product is of any real use.

Aminoguanidine

Aminoguanidine is one of the most promising anti-ageing drugs to be investigated in recent years, although it has been known about for some considerable time. We have already discussed the process of cross-linking or glycolysation of proteins by glucose molecules that causes an accumulation of AGEs (Advanced Glycation End products) – (*see* Carnosine, page 97). It is the acceleration of this process through the passage of time that is held to be responsible for much of the age-related damage seen in older age. The cross-linking process is even more marked in diabetes and it is believed that this is behind many of the complications seen in this disease.

The most important role of aminoguanidine is that it is able to inhibit the cross-linking process, and therefore reduce the damage that this can cause. More specifically, it has been shown to be beneficial in the treatment of heart and arterial disease, cataracts and glaucoma, to lower the level of harmful, low density lipoproteins (a damaging form of cholesterol) and to be helpful in lessening the effects and progression of kidney disease. Some anti-ageing specialists believe that aminoguanidine will prove to be useful in preventing and slowing down many other age-related effects as well, being supportive of the skin and all collagen-containing structures, bones, muscle, immune system and organ function.

Toxic side effects (nausea and headache) have been noted at higher doses in diabetic patients. However, a slightly lower dose removed these reactions and aminoguanidine is considered to be a safe and useful product by its supporters. As with most anti-ageing supplements, other scientists believe that this supplement is of little use.

Acetyl-L-Carnitine

Acetyl-L-Carnitine or ALC is the active form of the naturally occurring amino acid L-carnitine and is found in red meats, poultry, fish and dairy products. However, its supporters believe that it needs to be taken as a supplement in order to benefit from its anti-ageing properties. Its most important role is to act on the mitochondria of cells and to increase the amount of cellular energy available. This has wide ranging repercussions throughout the body, helping to protect cells against many forms of damage. In particular, ALC supplements have been shown to improve concentration and memory, protect the heart and circulation, strengthen muscles, boost the immune system and have a protective effect upon nerve cells. Its role in energy production and the utilisation of fats helps to regulate body weight. It has proved useful in the treatment of a number of age-related conditions including Parkinson's disease and Alzheimer's dementia. Some adverse side effects have been reported, particularly when the supplements are first taken and these include headaches, nausea and light-headedness. Supporters of ALC maintain that its benefits far outweigh any possible disadvantages while its detractors believe that it may not do any good or may even prove to be harmful.

Centrophenoxine

Centrophenoxine (Lucidril) is another anti-ageing supplement that has been studied extensively for many years and has been used clinically, although most evidence for its effectiveness has come from animal research. Centrophenoxine is a compound composed of two biochemical substances, dimethylamino-ethanol (DMAE) and parachlorophenoxyacetate (pCPA). DMAE is a naturally occurring substance within the body and is also found in protein foods, particularly fish and meat. DMAE is a source of choline that is vital for the production of neurotransmitters such as acetylcholine which are essential for the functioning of the brain and nervous system. It is on the brain and cognitive functions that centrophenoxine has its useful anti-ageing effects. During normal ageing, a biochemical waste pigment called lipofuscin accumulates within brain cells, adversely affecting their functioning and eventually causing cell death. Centrophenoxine is able to remove lipofuscin and hence helps to preserve brain cell function. It also has other powerful antioxidant activity within the brain and has been used to improve memory and intellectual functions in elderly people and those suffering from Alzheimer's dementia. A further benefit of centrophenoxine is that it stimulates protein synthesis within brain cells, aiding the physical repair of membranes and cellular components. It is believed that the pCPA component of centrophenoxine plays a role in this, along with DMAE.

In summary, centrophenoxine is said by its supporters to act as a brain 'energiser', slowing down and preventing the effects of ageing. Side effects (due to increased levels of acetylcholine) include headache, insomnia, irritability and hyperactivity but these are avoided at lower doses. People with Parkinson's disease and pregnant and nursing mothers should not take centrophenoxine and the drug should only be taken under medical supervision. Many scientists and clinicians would not support the use of centrophenoxine, especially in healthy people and the effects of long-term usage are not known.

Hydergine

Hydergine is another drug that has powerful effects upon the brain and belongs to a class of compounds known as ergotalkoloids. One of the most important ways in which hydergine operates involves its ability to protect the brain during periods of oxygen imbalance.

Oxygen is a 'double-edged sword' in the body – it is essential for life and yet it is also a source of free radical production. When plenty of oxygen is available, free radical production is cancelled out by oxygen's ability to neutralise them. However, during conditions of too much or too little oxygen, free radical production accelerates greatly. One of the main ways in which this happens is by a chemical reaction called peroxidation where oxygen reacts with unsaturated fats in cell membranes. Brain cells contain the highest proportion of unsaturated fats of any part of the body and hence are highly susceptible to oxygen-generated free radical damage. Eventually, this damage results in a disintegration of the membranes and death of the cells.

During ageing, atherosclerosis or hardening of the arteries often occurs, causing a decreased oxygen supply to tissues and organs with particular consequences for the brain. It is thought that the development of dementia, with all its consequent symptoms of irritability, short-term memory loss, confusion, etc. is possibly linked with declining oxygen supply.

Hydergine therapy, particularly at somewhat higher doses, significantly improves the mental functions of people with mild to moderate dementia and is a recognized treatment for this condition. It was thought that this improvement was brought about solely because hydergine enhances blood, and hence oxygen, supply to the brain. However, it has subsequently been discovered that hydergine benefits the brain in other ways as well. It can protect the brain from free radical damage during periods of oxygen imbalance, enhance the metabolic processes occurring within brain cells and promotes the formation of new nerve end connections – the dendrites. It is across the dendrites that one nerve cell passes messages (electrical impulses) to another and these connections are needed for correct nervous system function. Hydergine has also been shown to inhibit the accumulation of the waste pigment lipofuscin within brain cells and to promote the production and release of neurotransmitters.

Studies have also taken place to test the effects of hydergine upon the brain of healthy elderly people and some of these trials are still taking place. Early results indicate that hydergine may well act to preserve and protect brain function. Those receiving the treatment had higher and enhanced levels of electrical activity within the brain, lower blood cholesterol and showed improvement in heartbeat rate and circulation.

As well as being used as a treatment for dementia, many hospitals use hydergine to treat patients in life-threatening conditions of oxygen lack. Some also administer the drug before planned operations. Hydergine is not readily available and must be prescribed by a doctor. Many anti-ageing specialists believe that hydergine is set to become a major treatment to protect the brain in healthy people. Side effects appear to be few and slight, even with higher doses and longer term use, and are limited to nausea, slight digestive upsets and headaches, usually only in the short term.

Piracetam

Piracetam belongs to a class of drugs known as nootropics that are said to enhance the cognitive functions of the brain. Piracetam is biochemically similar to certain amino acids and is marketed under a considerable number of different trade names. It has been used to treat dementia and is said to improve memory, learning ability and concentration, although its mode of operation is not understood. It is believed that it has antioxidant properties and promotes blood flow and the transmission of information within the brain by being involved in complex metabolic processes. Piracetam is not commonly used in North America or in the UK but is prescribed in many European countries. Side effects are usually rare and short-lived and include digestive upsets and headaches. Research continues into the effects of piracetam with particular interest in its potential protective, anti-ageing capabilities.

Vinpocetine

Vinpocetine is an alkaloid drug produced by slightly altering an extract of the periwinkle plant known as vincamine. Vinpocetine acts specifically on the brain, boosting the cerebral metabolism in a number of beneficial ways. It boosts the conversion of glucose into energy and enhances the utilisation of glucose and energy by brain cells. It dilates cerebral blood vessels and enhances the elasticity of red blood cells which means that blood flows more easily through the brain, thereby increasing the amount of available oxygen. It affects the blood platelets (components that are involved in clotting) as well as the erythrocytes, making it less likely that clots will form and hence helping to reduce the risk of thrombosis and stroke. It has also been shown to protect the brain in conditions of oxygen lack.

Vinpocetine is used to improve memory, loss of speech or co-ordination, vertigo and dizziness resulting from problems with the organs of balance in the inner ear, anxiety, insomnia and glaucoma and eye conditions. It may help to improve intellectual and other disabilities resulting from stroke or circulatory disorders affecting the brain.

Some studies in healthy people have shown

improvements in cognitive functioning and memory following treatment with vinpocetine. The drug is generally considered to be safe and side effects are usually rare and short-lived. They include low blood pressure, feelings of weakness, raised heart beat rate, minor digestive upsets and a dry mouth. The drug should only be taken under medical supervision and it is considered that the best results are obtained by taking it for at least one year.

Nicotinamide

Nicotinamide adenine dinucleotide or NADH is a naturally occurring coenzyme, present in all cells in the body but with particular importance for the brain. A coenzyme is a substance that activates one or more enzymes – the protein catalysts necessary to set off metabolic reactions within living cells. Coenzymes are often the active form of vitamins. NADH is the active form of vitamin B_3. NADH plays a complex and vital role in all the cycles involved in the provision of energy within cells. It is manufactured within the body and also found in foods – particularly meat, chicken, fish and yeast. However, much of the NADH in food is lost for various reasons, before it can be used within the cells. Hence NADH needs to be taken in supplement form in order to gain its benefits.

As a result of ageing, the amount of energy available to the brain declines and it is believed that this is a factor in the development of conditions such as dementia and Parkinson's disease. A supplement of NADH was developed in the 1980s and clinical trials were conducted with people suffering from Alzheimer's disease. All patients showed significant improvements. Further tests were then carried out on people suffering from Parkinson's disease and age-related depression, and measurable improvements were once again seen. The results for Parkinson's disease were particularly encouraging as it is believed that NADH boosts the brain's own production of dopamine, something that is lacking in people with this disease and that conventional drug therapy has not been able to address.

Overall, NADH appears to have a positive effect (via complex biochemical interactions) on the production of the brain's own natural neurotransmitters, including dopamine and noradrenaline, as well as boosting energy availability. Further trials have been conducted that have shown that treatment with NADH is beneficial for those suffering from chronic fatigue syndrome. Several anti-ageing specialists believe that this natural substance may prevent the onset of age-related brain disorders. No adverse side effects have been reported and while many scientists remain sceptical, people using NADH continue to uphold its benefits.

S-Adenosyl L-Methionine

S-Adenosyl L-Methionine or SAMe is a natural substance, metabolised within the body from the amino acid (protein) methionine. Methionine itself is present in protein-rich foods such as meat, chicken and fish. A toxic waste product of methionine is the amino acid, homocysteine, which is now known to be involved in the development of heart disease and osteoporosis, inflammatory conditions and dementia. SAMe is synthesized by an enzymatic reaction that occurs primarily after dark and is linked with the operation of the internal biological clock (*see* melatonin, page 30, 153). During ageing, the level of SAMe declines and is mirrored by a rise in the amount of homocysteine.

SAMe is by far the most important participant in a process known as methylation, in which a methyl group (CH_2) is donated to another molecule, often DNA or a protein. Methylation is occurring all the time throughout life and is essential for many vital processes: the repair of DNA and the expression of genes, the action of hormones and neurotransmitters and the maintenance of the myelin sheath around nerves and repair of cartilage and joints. It is also involved in the removal of toxic waste products by the liver. Methylation cannot occur without SAMe which is also able to inactivate the toxic amino acid, homocysteine, described above. In conjunction with folic acid, vitamin B_{12} and zinc, SAMe is able to initiate a process that converts homocysteine into the valuable antioxidant, glutathione. Once the SAMe compound has donated its methyl group, it is still a useful source of other molecules such as sulphates.

SAMe has proved useful in the treatment of depression and it appears that it does this by acting on the receptor sites for brain neurotransmitters such as serotonin and dopamine, enhancing the mood altering effects of these natural chemicals. It has been shown to lessen pain in arthritis and to conserve and even improve the health of joint cartilage. In both these circumstances, SAMe has produced improvements without the side effects that can occur with conventional treatments. SAMe has proved useful in restoring liver function in people with damage sustained through drug or alcohol abuse (cirrhosis) or diseases such as hepatitis. This is due to the fact that SAMe has been shown to aid the liver in the removal of poisons.

The use of SAMe is still in its early stages and at present it is only prescribed in some countries for the treatment of depression. As levels of SAMe decline naturally with age, with adverse consequences for methylation and the protection of DNA, several specialists believe that this substance is set to become one of the key compounds for healthy ageing. Side effects are rare, generally short-lived and include digestive upset and nervousness. SAMe is now available in tablet form, although it remains fairly expensive.

Alternative and Complementary Therapies

S TRICTLY speaking, alternative therapies are those in which practitioners receive medical and clinical training and must pass exams before they are allowed to practise. Examples are osteopathy and chiropractic.

Complementary therapies include many other forms of healing in which practitioners have not necessarily received any medical training. In practice, however, most complementary therapists receive training and must complete courses in their chosen discipline in order to offer their services in that particular field.

However, complementary therapies must always aim to assist and support conventional medicine and never replace it. In recent years, there has been an enormous growth of interest in different forms of healing, not only amongst members of the public but from within the ranks of the medical profession. Many people are helped by these methods, which have the general advantage of being gentle forms of healing that do not produce adverse side effects. However, it is quite common for symptoms to initially get worse before any improvement is noted.

Alternative and complementary therapies can help in anti-ageing in several important ways: easing of pain and other symptoms in an age-related condition; relief of stress and anxiety and help with emotional problems; enhancing feelings of well-being or the belief that the healing process is being aided. This may support the immune system and the mind in the fight against a specific or more general age-related condition. Hence these therapies can assist the body's own inner healing resources.

Some of the therapies that may help with ageing are briefly described below and you may wish to find out more about one or some of them for yourself. However, if you have any particular symptoms or concerns, you should *always* first seek medical advice.

Acupuncture

Acupuncture is an ancient Chinese therapy that involves inserting needles into the skin at specific points of the body. Very fine, sterilised disposable needles are used and there should be no discomfort or pain. In modern practice, laser beams and electrical currents may be used to increase the effectiveness of the needles.

Western doctors believe that acupuncture may work through stimulating the neurosecretory cells to release natural pain killers – the endorphins. The

Chinese view is that the specific points of the body into which acupuncture needles are inserted are located along meridians – energy channels or pathways related to internal body organs. The energy is known as *qi* (*ch'i*) and the needles are manipulated to decrease or increase the flow or unblock it if it is impeded. Traditional Chinese medicine sees the body as being comprised of two natural, opposing but complementary forces known as yin and yang. Ailments and diseases are held to be caused by an imbalance of yin and yang that can be rectified by the use of acupuncture needles.

In the West, acupuncture has been used primarily to alleviate rheumatism, arthritis and back pain. However, it may help other disorders including stress, allergies, digestive problems and withdrawal symptoms (e.g. of someone giving up smoking).

Qualified acupuncturists complete three years training and belong to a professional association. However, anyone can use the title 'acupuncturist' so it is necessary to ensure that the person you consult has verifiable qualifications. Many GP practices now have arrangements with acupuncturists for referral of suitable patients.

Alexander technique

The Alexander technique is based on reacquiring good posture and correcting bad habits that, over many years, cause people to tense their bodies in an unnatural way, often resulting in pain and placing a strain on internal organs. The Alexander technique is completely harmless and encourages an equitable state between mind and body. A practitioner helps a client to relax and release muscular tension (possibly by using some gentle manipulation or positioning) and assists the person to gradually learn to 'flow' and move more effectively, with minimum effort. With practice, correct use of the body can be achieved and become natural to that person. The technique benefits people of all ages and has been found to help athletes, dancers, actors and public speakers.

A number of ailments may be relieved including depression, stress, headaches, anxiety, asthma, high blood pressure, respiratory problems, arthritis, sciatica and peptic ulcer.

Aromatherapy

Aromatherapy is a method of healing using very concentrated essential oils that are often highly aromatic and are extracted from plants. Different parts of the same plant may produce their own form of oil and these are extracted by a special process. Essential oils used in aromatherapy tend to be costly as vast quantities of plant material are used to extract them by a series of complex processes. The oils have healing properties – something that has been recognized since ancient times – and they have a very long history of use.

Essential oils are highly concentrated, volatile and aromatic and readily change, evaporate and deteriorate if exposed to light, heat and air. For most purposes in aromatherapy, essential oils are used in dilute form, being added either to water or to another oil called the base or carrier. These mixtures have a short shelf life of two or three months and so they are usually mixed at the time of use, in small amounts.

Various techniques are used in aromatherapy, of which massage is the most familiar. Essential oils pass through the skin and are taken into the body, exerting healing and beneficial effects upon internal tissues and organs. The oils used for massage should always have been mixed with a base and an aromatherapist will design an individual mixture, based upon a detailed client history.

Adding drops of an essential oil to bathwater is another way of achieving some of the beneficial effects of aromatherapy. It is soothing and relaxing, eases aches and pains, and the vapours are inhaled as they evaporate from the hot water. Inhalation is thought to be the most direct and rapid means of treatment. This is because the molecules of the volatile essential oil act directly on the olfactory organs and are immediately perceived by the brain. Inhalation can be carried out by adding one or two drops of an oil to a bowl of boiling water and then placing one's face above and over the bowl while surrounding the head with a towel.

Aromatherapy oils can be used in the home but people with asthma, high blood pressure, allergic skin conditions and pregnant women should exercise caution. A wide range of conditions and disorders may benefit from aromatherapy including arthritis, rheumatic and digestive complaints, throat, mouth and urinary tract infections, headaches, high blood pressure, skin complaints, menopausal symptoms and circulatory disorders. Therapists believe that aromatherapy can be preventative and protective with regard to some illnesses and age-related conditions.

Autogenic training

Autogenic training is a form of therapy that seeks to teach a person to relax, thereby relieving stress. This is achieved by learning a series of six basic exercises that can be undertaken either lying flat, sitting in an armchair or sitting on the edge of a chair with the head bent forward and the chin on the chest. By learning the techniques and exercises of autogenic training, a person is able to achieve a state of relaxation and tranquillity, sleep more restfully and generally has more energy and a greater feeling of well-being. Autogenic training is taught in small group sessions and may be available on the NHS as well as privately.

Ayurvedic medicine

Ayurvedic medicine is an Indian, holistic form of therapy that is gaining an increasing number of followers in western countries. Preventative measures and the maintenance of good health is very much a part of the Ayurvedic philosophy that holds that life is governed by three forces, each controlling a number of different functions. A practitioner obtains a detailed picture of every aspect of his patient's life and may advocate a particular form of treatment in the event of any changes, even if no symptoms of disorder are present.

Methods of treatment include a great variety of medicines that are derived from plant and mineral sources, meditation, yoga and other exercises, religious ceremonies, water and steam baths, massage and particular diets. Ayurvedic treatments are derived from centuries of use and work for very many people, although many have not been subjected to rigorous scientific trials. The emphasis on prevention is one of the main strengths of this form of therapy and makes it eminently suitable for anti-ageing. The fact that the practitioner and patient must necessarily develop a close working relationship no doubt proves helpful and provides reassurance for those seeking Ayurvedic treatment.

Bach flower remedies

Bach remedies consist of 38 preparations derived from floating freshly-picked flowers on spring water. Drops of the diluted remedies are then used to treat a number of different emotional and physical conditions. Bach remedies are entirely gentle and safe and can be used by people of all ages on a self-help basis. Although there is no known scientific reason for their effectiveness, very many people find relief and are helped by them. They are well worth trying on the understanding that they may help and will certainly not cause harm.

Chiropractic

Chiropractic is used to relieve pain by manipulation, mainly of the spine, to correct any problems that are present. Misalignment of the spine can cause widespread problems not merely confined to the back. However, dealing with back pain, which is very much connected with ageing, forms a large part of the chiropractor's work. Doctors are increasingly recognizing the value of chiropractic for treating back problems but would probably be less sure about its wider role. Most people acquire irregularities in the spine and sometimes this begins in infancy or childhood. Chiropractic can help many people, sometimes in unexpected ways, but it is essential to find a properly qualified practitioner if you are considering this form of therapy.

Colour therapy

Colour therapy uses coloured light to treat disease

and disorder and to help restore good health. It is well known that human beings respond to coloured light and are affected by rays of various wavelengths. This even occurs in people who are blind, proving that the human body is able to respond in subtle ways to electromagnetic radiation. Colour therapists believe that part of this response involves each person emitting a unique pattern of colours or aura that can be recorded by a method known as Kirlian photography. Disturbances in the pattern of the aura indicate the presence of disorder or disease.

Treatment consists of bathing the body in an appropriate combination of coloured light, determined by the therapist. The aim is to restore the natural balance in the pattern of the aura. Almost any condition can be treated by this method. In orthodox medicine it is accepted that colours exert subtle influences on people particularly upon their mood and psychological well-being.

Colour therapy may well aid healing, even in the absence of scientific explanation and is a gentle, safe form of treatment.

Herbal remedies
Herbal medicine can be viewed as the precursor of modern pharmacology and it continues today as an effective and natural method of treating and preventing illness. As such, it is eminently suitable for use in

anti-ageing. The medicinal use of herbs is aid to be as old as mankind and the earliest records date back to 1500 BC and late Egyptian civilisation. Even then, herbal practice was hundreds of years old and its record of efficacy not only spans the centuries but every country and culture as well. Globally, herbal medicine is three to four times more commonly practised than conventional medicine.

Herbs are organic and not man-made, synthetic substances, and so possess an affinity for the human organism. They can be used to treat an enormous range of conditions and disorders and can help to restore a sense of well-being and relaxation necessary to the support of the body's own defences against disease. The choice of treatment should ideally be based upon a thorough health assessment and the experience and training of a qualified practitioner. However, many remedies are now available from chemists and health stores, etc. and large numbers of people opt for self-treatment. Care must be taken if this is the case as some herbs are potent and can cause side effects. Also, they may react with conventional drugs and so you should not use herbal remedies with prescription medication without your doctor's approval. This is particularly the case with Chinese herbs, some of which can be dangerous. The origins of others may be dubious in that they may contain impurities.

Homeopathy

Homeopathy is one of the most familiar of the alternative therapies and is widely used alongside conventional medicine. The approach is holistic with the overall state of health of the patient, especially his or her psychological and emotional well-being, regarded as being highly significant. A homeopathic remedy must be suitable both for the symptoms and the characteristics and temperament of the patient. Hence two patients with the same illness may be offered different remedies suited to their individual natures. Likewise, one remedy may be used to treat different groups of symptoms or ailments.

Homeopathic remedies are based on the concept that 'like cures like', an ancient philosophy that was revived in the 19th century. They are derived from plant, animal and mineral sources. Substances used are first soaked in alcohol to extract their essential ingredients and to produce a solution called the 'Mother Tincture'. This is then diluted several times, with the more dilute remedies being held to have greater potency. The remedies are made into tablets or they may be used in the form of ointment, solutions, powders, suppositories, etc. High potency (i.e. more dilute) remedies are used for severe symptoms.

It is widely accepted that homeopathic remedies are safe and non-addictive – even the more concentrated ones contain infinitesimal quantities of the original substance. Some homeopathic remedies are now sold in chemists and health shops for self-treatment, but it is best to consult a qualified homeopath (some of whom are medical doctors) in order to obtain the best individual treatment. Homeopathy is a gentle therapy, suitable for all age groups and for many ailments and conditions, including those related to ageing.

Hydrotherapy

Hydrotherapy is the use of water to heal and ease a variety of ailments, either as hot or cool baths or showers, steam or sitz baths, wrapping or ice packs. The relaxing and pain-relieving effects of a hot bath are known to everyone but other hydrotherapy techniques are perhaps less familiar. Hydrotherapy must be used cautiously in the elderly, the very young and those with certain conditions and illnesses. Its main benefits are in the treatment of chronic pain, as in arthritis and rheumatism, boosting the immune system (which is vital for anti-ageing), stimulating the circulation and for the relief of stress and anxiety.

Laughter therapy

The good news about laughter therapy is that it is fun and can be practised anytime, anywhere! You may laugh alone or in company and if, at first, you feel inhibited, try smiling instead. Hearty laughter relieves stress and depression, enhances the sense of well-being and is even a form of aerobic exercise – all of which are anti-ageing!

Massage

Massage or rubbing a painful area of the body is a natural response in human beings. Therapeutic massage, often incorporating the use of perfumed oils, was used as long ago as 3000 BC and it forms a part of several other therapies. Today, it is used to achieve relaxation and relief of mental and physical stress and strain that often results in muscular aches and pains. It is also useful for the treatment of headaches, high blood pressure, insomnia, sinusitis and hyperactivity and helps to boost the circulation and immune system. Massage promotes a feeling of calmness and well-being that is especially helpful for people prone to bouts of mild depression. Various techniques are used and the therapeutic value of massage is well recognized by conventional medical practitioners.

Naturopathy

As the name suggests, naturopathy very much depends upon nature and natural things and is a holistic philosophy that is not only an approach to healing but a way of life. Of fundamental importance is the fact that naturopathy is concerned as much with disease prevention as with cure and so it is an extremely suitable approach with regard to ageing. Naturopathy has several key elements. These are: nutrition and diet, including the use of vitamin and mineral supplements when necessary; detoxification – the use of short periods of fasting or controlled diets and supplements to aid the natural elimination of toxic substances; hydrotherapy; herbal remedies; stress control and relaxation; exercise; other alternative therapies, and lifestyle counselling.

It can be seen that the full scope of naturopathy is extremely broad and most practitioners develop a particular area of interest. A naturopath will always wish to obtain a detailed history of the client before recommending any particular course of action. The naturopathic approach is based on sound principles and is a gentle therapy that is particularly suitable for the relief and prevention of age-related problems.

Osteopathy

Osteopathy is a technique that uses manipulation and massage to help correct problems in the spine, joints and muscles to make them work smoothly and effectively once again. Almost everyone develops or sustains some degree of skeletal, joint or muscle damage as a result of ageing. Or a trauma or accident may be the initial cause and sometimes this can be an old injury that sets up problems in middle or older age. The physical misalignment may itself cause pain or it may cause the person unconsciously to hold himself in a certain way or to clench muscles in order to compensate. Eventually this results in pain, possibly in an area removed from the site of the problem. Clenching muscles and becoming tense as a result of psychological stress can itself cause problems to bones and joints, especially if prolonged. Most people who seek the services of an osteopath do so because of pain that is often severe and frequently related to a disorder in the back. After careful examination, the osteopath manipulates and massages the joints, spine and muscles to correct any misalignment and to bring about relief of pain.

There are many other complementary therapies that may be helpful for individual people in the prevention and treatment of particular conditions. It is impossible to describe them all here but if you are interested, information is readily available on most forms of alternative treatment. However, the more unusual therapies may not necessarily be available in your area and, of course, the cost of all these treatments is something that must always be taken into account.

Conditions and Treatments

Selected examples of age-related conditions with suggested anti-ageing treatments

Alzheimer's dementia

Alzheimer's disease is the commonest cause of dementia among the elderly and is a degenerative disease of the cerebral cortex of the brain. It is caused by the build-up of abnormal, waste material within cells. The disease is progressive and sufferers may exhibit a range of symptoms such as short-term memory loss, confusion, inability to concentrate, irritability and inattention to personal hygiene. In severe cases, the person may eventually fail to recognize family members, suffer a personality change or lose the power of speech and become incontinent. There is no cure but some drug treatments that boost the availability of natural neurochemicals may help. Other therapies that can help are reminiscence about the past, music to stimulate memory, playing card and board games to get the mind working, etc. and these are often the approaches that are used in residential care homes for the elderly. Attention to diet is important, with supplements of vitamins and minerals, if necessary. As discussed in earlier sections, many dietary elements are protective of the brain and these are particularly important for a person with Alzheimer's disease. Supplements that may help include vitamins B and E, selenium, coenzyme Q_{10}, Ginkgo biloba, carnosine, phospholipids, HGH, pregnenolone, gerovital, acetyl-L-carnitine, centrophenoxine, hydergine, piracetam, NADH and SAMe.

Arterial disease – atherosclerosis and heart disease

Some degeneration of the arteries is almost certainly an inevitable consequence of ageing, but should not normally have adverse consequences. However, atherosclerosis – a degenerative disease in which fatty deposits build up on arterial walls, leading to a narrowing of the internal diameter and hence reduced blood flow – is very much linked to a western diet and lifestyle.

A high consumption of saturated (animal) fat and salt, low consumption of fruit, vegetables and fibre and lack of exercise mean that the early signs of atherosclerosis are increasingly being detected in children. This is causing a great deal of concern since atherosclerosis is very much linked with the occurrence of thrombosis, heart attack and stroke. It is feared that these often fatal conditions will increasingly affect younger adults, unless the situation can be improved. Atherosclerosis and heart disease are very much linked together in western countries. Heart disease may take several different forms but a high proportion of its incidence is regarded as preventable. The major risk factors for both atherosclerosis and heart disease are, first and foremost, smoking, poor diet, obesity and lifestyle factors such as lack of exercise and stress.

Giving up smoking, adopting a good healthy diet that is protective of the heart and circulation, losing excess weight, taking regular, aerobic exercise and tackling stress are the key measures to take in order to reduce individual risk. Supplements that may help include coenzyme Q_{10} and SAMe (which removes the dangerous amino acid homocysteine that is implicated in the development of atherosclerosis and heart disease). Many people take half an aspirin or a junior aspirin each day as this helps to thin the blood and reduce the risk of clotting. However, this should be used cautiously, since aspirin can cause bleeding in the digestive tract in susceptible people and it is best to first seek medical advice. Many complementary therapies are supportive of the heart and arteries either directly, as with some herbal remedies, or indirectly, through measures that combat stress, lower blood pressure and promote an efficient circulation.

Diabetes mellitus

Diabetes occurs in two forms that produce similar symptoms and problems but only one form is related to ageing.

Essentially, diabetes is a complex metabolic disorder involving the energy molecule, glucose, which is mainly derived from carbohydrates in foods but also from fats and proteins. In diabetes, there is an accumulation of glucose in the blood caused by a lack of the vital hormone, insulin, produced by cells in the pancreas. The glucose is not broken down to release energy but instead, builds up in the blood causing hyperglycaemia. It is also excreted by the kidneys. (An important test for diabetes is to measure the amount of glucose present in urine). Early symptoms of diabetes include excessive thirst, frequent urination, tiredness, recurrent infections and weight loss. If the condition remains untreated, further severe symptoms can develop that in the worst cases include convulsions and coma.

One form of diabetes, called insulin-dependent diabetes mellitus, or IDDM, usually appears in childhood and used to be called juvenile-onset diabetes. As the name implies, IDDM requires treatment with insulin, given by self-administered injections and careful attention to diet. A second type of diabetes more commonly develops in older people. It is called non-insulin-dependent diabetes mellitus or NIDDM and was formerly referred to as maturity-onset diabetes. This type affects 15% of all people aged over 50 but the true incidence may be higher as evidence suggests that it is frequently undiagnosed. This is a worrying situation since untreated diabetes, in particular, carries with it a number of potentially serious health risks. Anyone with diabetes has an increased risk of eventually developing eye and kidney problems, arterial and heart disease but with care these can be minimised and controlled. NIDDM can sometimes be treated by means of diet alone, depending upon severity, but other cases may need insulin.

Whether insulin is needed or not, diet is critical in the management of diabetes. Fortunately, the advice is the same as that for healthy eating, i.e. a diet based on complex carbohydrates that are high in starch and fibre and provide a slow release of energy, thus avoiding 'peaks' of blood glucose. Refined sugar in any form should mostly be avoided although somewhat ironically, in the case of a hypoglycaemic attack, glucose or sucrose is precisely what is needed.

Hypoglycaemia or low blood sugar is a condition that mainly affects people receiving insulin although it is a risk for any diabetic. It occurs because of an imbalance between the dose of insulin injected and the amount of carbohydrate eaten, resulting in too little glucose in the blood. This explains why many diabetics have to carefully monitor their food intake and may need to eat small amounts frequently. Sufferers often become adept at recognizing the early symptoms of hypoglycaemia, which include light-headedness, weakness, sweating and confusion and can remedy the situation by taking glucose by mouth. Without treatment, the person becomes increasingly disturbed and may slip into unconsciousness and coma. (It is always worth remembering that someone who appears to be drunk may, in fact, be having a hypoglycaemic attack).

Emergency medical help should be summoned as the patient will require glucose by injection to effect a recovery. Anyone who is susceptible to hypoglycaemia usually wears a special bracelet or carries a card so that others can be alerted.

In order to lessen the risk of developing NIDDM, sugar intake should be kept low and a healthy diet eaten throughout life. It is important to lose weight if overweight or obese. The increased incidence of NIDDM is directly connected with rising levels of obesity. People over the age of 50 are advised to have regular blood tests since the onset of NIDDM is often insidious and passes unnoticed.

Many foods and natural substances are helpful for diabetes, both directly and indirectly (i.e. by supporting tissues and organs that may be at risk of damage arising from diabetes-related conditions). Alternative therapies can likewise be helpful both in prevention and treatment. Useful supplements include the hormone DHEA and aminoguanidine but these treatments are unlikely to be endorsed by medical professionals.

Eye problems – cataract and Age-related Macular Degeneration (ARMD)

Cataract is a condition where the lens of the eye becomes opaque, resulting in blurring of vision. It may have a number of different causes, including diabetes, but is most commonly produced by changes in the protein components of the lens as a consequence of ageing. Free radical damage and a lifetime's exposure to sunlight (ultraviolet radiation) are believed to contribute to the development of cataracts. Research suggests that a high consumption of carotenoids may be protective and it is obviously sensible to wear a hat and sunglasses to protect the eyes. Alternative therapies, particularly naturopathy, may be helpful. None of the known anti-ageing supplements directly affect the lens but some may be generally supportive of the health of the eyes.

Age-related macular degeneration concerns a part of the retina – the layer that lines the interior of the eye that contains light sensitive cells and on which an image is formed. The macula lutea is a yellowish-coloured, oval-shaped spot on the retina on which the sharpest, central part of an image is formed. Degeneration of this area is a common cause of partial blindness, often leading to a blurring of central vision while that at the periphery remains unaffected. Causes are unclear but it is believed that free radical damage and sunlight are involved and smokers are also much more likely to be affected. People with brown eyes are less susceptible. As with cataract, a diet high in carotenoids and isoflavones is recommended and selenium and zinc supplements may be helpful. Naturopathic and herbal remedies, among the complementary therapies may also be generally supportive of the health of the eyes.

Osteoarthritis

This is the most common form of arthritis in those in middle and older age and it is believed that most people over the age of 50 show some signs of this condition. Osteoarthritis is a degeneration of joint cartilage with accompanying changes in the bone. It usually involves the loss of cartilage and the development of osteophytes (abnormal bony projections) at the bone margins. The function of the joint (most commonly the thumb, spine, knee and hip) is affected and it becomes swollen and painful. Early symptoms include stiffness upon rising in the morning or following rest. Conventional treatment relies upon anti-inflammatory and analgesic drugs and replacement surgery, in severe cases. The latter is usually a very successful treatment but the surgery sometimes needs to be repeated.

There are several ways in which an individual can try and prevent the onset of this condition. It is important to maintain a healthy weight as it is obvious that any excess is going to put a constant strain on joints. It is also vital is to remain active and to take regular exercise, preferably in a variety of forms so that the joints are kept mobile in different ways. Once again, diet is vital in the fight against osteoarthritis and it is wise to regularly eat oily fish and plenty of anti-oxidant-rich fruits and vegetables. Helpful anti-ageing supplements are glucosamine and chondroitin and many arthritis sufferers take these, to beneficial effect. More controversial supplements for osteoarthritis include SAMe, pregnenolone and DHEA. There are many complementary therapies that may be helpful including naturopathy and hydrotherapy, herbal remedies (capsaicin, devil's claw, aloe vera, feverfew, bogbean, ginger root and others), homeopathy (arnica and rhus tox), massage, osteopathy, chiropractic and acupuncture. Using some of these should hopefully ease the condition but anyone suffering from arthritis should always seek medical advice.

Osteoporosis

Osteoporosis is a loss of bone tissue so that the bones become thin and brittle and susceptible to fractures. Calcium and other minerals are lost and also the protein and collagen components that form the matrix of the bone. The condition is common in post-menopausal women and is related to the decline in the hormone, oestrogen, which is protective before the menopause. Long-term use of steroidal drugs can also be a cause and the condition may affect men. In general, men are less susceptible because they have a greater initial density of bone and a more robust skeleton.

In youth and before the age of 30, the bones store calcium, which is then used for maintenance and repair. Beyond this age, the stores are gradually depleted as they are used at a faster rate than that at which they are replenished. It is extremely important to eat plenty of calcium-rich foods in youth to ensure that the bones have a plentiful store of this essential mineral to cope with this natural decline.

The process of change in bone density begins quite early in life with the gradual loss of calcium. However, this is not osteoporosis as the bones at this stage remain strong. Osteoporosis describes a far more marked state of loss of several of the components of bone. For women, the menopause is significant because the fall in oestrogen levels accelerates the loss of calcium, and their bones are naturally lighter and less dense than those of men. The causes of osteoporosis in men are less clear but in elderly people of both sexes, the symptoms are similar. These include pain, especially in the back with the possible development of curvature of the spine, loss of height and fractures that may result from a relatively minor accident. Often, the first diagnosis of osteoporosis is made when an elderly person is admitted to hospital with a fracture – commonly of the hip, wrist or spine.

There are a number of diagnostic tests that can be performed to ascertain the state of the bones and whether osteoporosis is present.

In conventional medicine, hormone replacement therapy (HRT) during and after the menopause is known to be effective and protective for women in reducing the risk of osteoporosis. Of course, this hormonal treatment can also help to relieve menopausal symptoms. A newer group of drugs, which are not hormones, are the SERMs (selective oestrogen receptor modulators) which balance the fluctuating levels of oestrogen during the menopause. These may be used more widely in the future and are protective of the bones without the possible drawbacks of HRT.

For those who do not wish to take synthetic hormones, there are herbal remedies called phytoestrogens, and others called natural progesterones, which have hormonal activity. These include black cohosh, false unicorn root, liquorice, fennel, ginseng and dong quai. However, it is essential to use these only under qualified supervision as, contrary to popular belief, these are powerful substances that may produce unwanted side effects. They are usually used to combat menopausal symptoms, but may be protective of the bones as well.

Two major lifestyle factors are important in preventing and treating osteoporosis and these are, as we have seen, diet and exercise. Not only should the diet contain calcium-rich foods such as low fat dairy products, but also plentiful fruits, vegetables, nuts, seeds and berries which are abundant sources of antioxidants and flavonoids. Phytoestrogens can be obtained from foods, especially soya, chick peas and other pulses and nuts. (Food sources do not produce any adverse effects). The utilisation of calcium within the body is significant in osteoporosis, and other vitamins and minerals are also important. These include vitamins D, B_6, B_{12}, K, folic acid, magnesium, zinc, boron and strontium. The diet should include foods containing all of these but middle-aged women are advised to take calcium and magnesium supplements (each in the form of citrate) to ensure that they have a plentiful supply.

One of the reasons why exercise is so vital throughout life is to preserve the strength of the bones. Brisk walking, dancing, skipping, jumping and weight-bearing exercises pump calcium into the bones and help it to stay there! You may not have the time (or the money) to visit a gym with specialized weight-lifting equipment but you can improvise at home, using books, bags of sugar or flour, etc! People who perform such exercises regularly have been shown to have stronger bones than those who do not. Also, at any age, the condition of the bones can be improved with appropriate exercise. However, anyone with existing osteoporosis or who is elderly, should not exercise without seeking medical advice and must be careful to avoid falls and accidents. Yoga, T'ai-Chi

Ch'uan and other Oriental forms of exercise are also suitable in the prevention and treatment of osteoporosis.

Medical treatment for established osteoporosis sometimes involves the use of drugs called biphosphonates which act directly on bone to increase its strength. These are used particularly for people who are considered to be at risk of fractures and many elderly people with osteoporosis are now in receipt of medication for this condition. Among the anti-ageing supplements, SAMe, regeneressen and aminoguanidine have been shown to be helpful in some cases of osteoporosis, as are many of the complementary therapies.

Prostate gland enlargement – Benign Prostatic Hypertrophy (BPH)

The prostate is a small gland of the male reproductive system that is located below the bladder and which opens into the urethra. It contributes an alkaline fluid into semen that assists the movement of sperm. Benign prostatic hypertrophy is an enlargement of the gland that is a common condition in older men. The operation of the gland is governed by complex hormonal factors and it is possible that imbalances in these may be responsible for BPH, which causes problems because of the gland's close proximity to the bladder. The condition causes pressure to be exerted on the neck of the bladder, obstructing the flow of urine. The bladder consequently extends and there is a frequent need to pass urine, especially during the night, but often a poor stream or spraying, dribbling and discomfort or pain. Continual sleep disturbance is one of the most wearing factors of this condition.

Since the bladder is not being emptied effectively, there is an increased risk of infection that can, in severe cases, involve the upper urinary tract and kidneys. A man with symptoms of BPH should always have medical investigations to rule out a less common cause of these symptoms which is prostatic cancer. When BPH is diagnosed, it is usual in conventional medicine to try drug treatments in the first instance, particularly if the symptoms are not too severe. Drugs may act to relax the muscles within the prostate, so relieving the pressure on the bladder, or to reduce the size of the gland itself. Eventually, and in severe cases of BPH surgical removal of the gland (prostatectomy) may become necessary. This is usually a very successful treatment but it can cause some subsequent problems relating to sexual performance.

Naturopathy and herbal remedies offer alternatives for both the prevention and treatment of prostate gland problems. There is a suspicion among naturopaths that the increasingly common incidence of BPH may be related to high levels of pollutants, such as heavy metals and pesticide residues in the environment. These pollutants can be detected in the tissues of people in western countries and many of them are ingested in food. Eating a wholefood diet (as far as possible from organic sources) that is rich in fibre, vitamins, minerals, flavonoids and carotenoids aids the body's natural detoxification processes and lowers blood cholesterol levels. (Accumulation of cholesterol and its metabolic products within the gland is believed to be a factor in the development of BPH). Oily fish and vegetable oils should be included. Vitamin and mineral supplements including B_6 and zinc, and evening primrose, sunflower, linseed, walnut and soya oils can improve symptoms in some patients.

The most important herbal remedy is undoubtedly an extract derived from the berries of a type of dwarf palm tree, saw palmetto. This extract has been shown to block the action of an enzyme that converts the hormone testosterone into a different form, dihydrotestosterone. Dihydrotestosterone stimulates the growth and enlargement of prostatic cells and by its action saw palmetto reduces this process.

Several studies have shown that the extract can significantly improve the symptoms in some sufferers, and with few or no side effects compared to conventional drugs. The only side effect that has (rarely) been reported is slight digestive upset and the extract works best in men with mild symptoms. Anti-ageing specialists may recommend saw palmetto as a preventative against prostate problems for older men but, in general, conventional medicine remains sceptical about its use. Herbalists may also recommend other remedies for prostate problems including ginseng, nettle root, African plum, couch grass, horsetail and African star grass. Most of these are held to have diuretic properties and act to support bladder function.

Other complementary therapies include hydrotherapy (especially sitz baths and hot and cold showering), homeopathy (pulsatilla, apis mel, belladonna) and acupuncture.

Glossary of Terms

This glossary contains selected terms to provide a quick reference to technical and/or medical words in the text.

alkaloid organic compounds which give medicinal properties to many drugs. Alkaloids occur mainly in flowering plants and many are derived from pyridine, quinoline and related compounds. They include several important drugs, such as morphine, quinine, caffeine and cocaine.

amino acids the end products of the digestion of protein foods and the building blocks from which all the protein components of the body are built up. They contain an acidic carboxyl group (-COOH) and an amino group (-NH₂), which are both bonded to the same central carbon atom. Some can be manufactured within the body whereas others, the essential amino acids, must be derived from protein sources in the diet.

antibiotic a substance, derived from a microorganism, that kills or inhibits the multiplication of other microorganisms, usually bacteria or fungi. Well known examples are penicillin and streptomycin.

antibodies protein substances of the globulin type which are produced by the lymphoid tissue and circulate in the blood. They react with their corresponding antigens and neutralize them. Antibodies are produced against a wide variety of antigens. These reactions are responsible for immunity and allergy.

antioxidant in molecules and cells, antioxidants deactivate free radicals that are the natural by-products of many cellular processes. Free radicals are also created by exposure to various environmental agents such as tobacco smoke and radiation. They can cause damage to cell components that over time may lead to diseases such as cancer. Antioxidants neutralise the free radicals before damage can be done.

arthritis inflammation of the joints or spine, the symptoms of which are pain and swelling, restriction of movement, redness and warmth of the skin. There are many different causes of arthritis, including osteoarthritis, rheumatoid arthritis, tuberculosis and rheumatic fever.

atheroma a degenerative condition of the arteries. The inner and middle coats of the arterial walls become scarred, and fatty deposits (cholesterol) are built up at these sites. The blood circulation is impaired, which may lead to such problems as angina pectoris, stroke and heart attack. The condition is associated with the western lifestyle, i.e. lack of exercise, smoking, obesity and too high an intake of animal fats.

atherosclerosis similar to atheroma, being a degenerative disease of the arteries associated with fatty deposits on the inner walls leading to reduced blood flow.

ATP *abbreviation for* adenosine triphosphate, an important molecule that is used as energy to drive all cellular processes. ATP can be synthesized during glycolysis, or it can be broken down to form ADP. This releases energy that will be used to drive a metabolic process, such as active transport across cell membranes or the contraction of muscle cells.

bacteria (*sing* **bacterium**) single celled organisms that underpin all life-sustaining processes. They are identified by shape: spiral, (spirilli), rod-like (bacilli), spherical (cocci), comma-shaped (vibrios) and the spirochaetal, which are corkscrew-like. Bacteria are the key agents in the chemical cycles of carbon, oxygen, nitrogen and sulphur.

B-cells these are lymphocytes, which differentiate in the bone marrow to form part of the immune system of humans. B-cells become activated when they encounter a specific antigen, leading to proliferation and secretion of antibodies by the activated B-cells. After a first encounter with an antigen, some of the B-cells remain and serve as memory cells. The memory cells will be capable of recognizing the same antigen during any subsequent encounter and will therefore produce a faster and greater secondary response (this is the principle behind vaccination).

cartilage a type of firm connective tissue that is pliable and forms part of the skeleton. There are three different kinds: hyaline cartilage, fibrocartilage and elastic cartilage. Hyaline cartilage is found at the joints of movable bones, in the trachea, nose and bronchi, and as costal cartilage joining the ribs to the breast bone. Fibrocartilage, which consists of cartilage and connective tissue, is found in the intervertebral discs of the spinal column and in tendons. Elastic cartilage is found in the external part of the ear (pinna).

cholesterol a fatty insoluble molecule which is widely found in the body and is synthesized from saturated fatty acids in the liver. Cholesterol is an important substance in the body. It is a component of cell membranes and a precursor in the production of steroid hormones (sex hormones) and bile salts. An elevated level of blood cholesterol is associated with atheroma, which may result in high blood pressure and coronary thrombosis, which is seen in the disease diabetes mellitus. It is generally recommended that people should reduce their consumption of saturated fat and look for alternatives in the form of unsaturated fats, which are found in vegetable oils.

chromosomes the rod-like structures, present in the nucleus of every body cell, that carry genetic information or genes. Each human body cell contains 23 pairs of chromosomes (apart from the sperm and ova), half derived from the mother and half from the father. Each chromosome consists of a coiled double filament (double helix) of DNA, with genes carrying the genetic information in linear form along its length. The genes determine all the characteristics of each individual. 22

of the chromosome pairs are the same in males and females. The 23rd pair are the sex chromosomes. Males have one X and one Y, whereas females have two X-chromosomes.

diabetes mellitus a complex metabolic disorder involving carbohydrate, fat and protein. It is the result of a lack of insulin produced by the pancreas, so that sugars are not broken down to release energy. This results in an accumulation of sugar in the blood and urine. Fats are thus used as an alternative energy source. Symptoms include thirst, polyuria and loss of weight, and the use of fats can produce ketosis and ketonuria. In its severest form, convulsions are followed by a diabetic coma.

Treatment relies on dietary control with doses of insulin or drugs. Long-term effects include thickening of the arteries, and in some cases the eyes, kidneys, nervous system, skin and circulation may be affected.

diphtheria an infectious disease caused by the bacterium *Corynebacterium diphtheriae* and commonest in children. The infection causes a membranous lining on the throat, which can interfere with breathing and eating. The toxin produced by the bacterium damages heart tissue and the central nervous system, and it can be fatal if not treated. The infection is countered by injection of antitoxin with penicillin or erythromycin given to kill the bacterium. Diphtheria can be prevented by vaccination.

diverticulosis the condition in which there are diverticula (*see* DIVERTICULUM) in the large intestine, occurring primarily in the lower colon. They are caused by the muscles of the bowel forcing the bowel out through weak points in the wall. It is thought that it may be related to diet. Symptoms are not always produced.

diverticulum (*pl* **diverticula**) in general, a pouch extending from a main cavity. Specifically, in the intestine, a sac-like protrusion through the wall, many of which usually develop later in life and are thought to be related to dietary factors. The formation of diverticula is called diverticulosis, and their inflammation is called diverticulitis.

DNA (**deoxyribonucleic acid**) a nucleic acid and the primary constituent of chromosomes. It transmits genetic information from parents to offspring in the form of genes. It is a very large molecule comprising two twisted nucleotide chains that can store enormous amounts of information in a stable but not rigid way, i.e. parental traits and characteristics are passed on but evolutionary changes are allowed to occur.

electron an indivisible particle that is negatively charged and free to orbit the positively charged nucleus of every atom. In the traditional model, electrons move around in concentric shells. However, the latest concept, based on quantum mechanics, regards the electron moving around the nucleus in clouds that can assume various shapes, such as a dumb-bell (two electrons moving) or clover leaf (four moving electrons). The shape and density of the outermost electronic shell will help determine what reactions are possible between particular atoms and molecules, e.g. whether an atom will easily gain or lose electrons to form an ion.

endocrine glands ductless glands that produce hormones for secretion directly into the bloodstream or lymph. Some organs, e.g. the pancreas, also release secretions via a duct. In addition to the pancreas, the major endocrine glands are the thyroid, pituitary, parathyroid, ovary and testis. Imbalances in the secretions of endocrine glands produce a variety of diseases.

enzyme any protein molecule that acts as a catalyst in the biochemical processes of the body. They are essential to life and are highly specific, acting on certain substrates at a set temperature and pH. Examples are the digestive enzymes amylase, lipase and trypsin. Enzymes act by providing active sites (one or more for each enzyme) to which substrate molecules bind, forming a short-lived intermediate. The rate of reaction is increased, and after the product is formed, the active site is freed. Enzymes are easily rendered inactive by heat and some chemicals. Enzymes are vital for the normal functioning of the body, and their lack or inactivity can produce metabolic disorders.

erythroblast a cell occurring in the red bone marrow that develops into a red blood cell (erythrocyte). The cell is colourless at first but accumulates haemoglobin and becomes red. In mammals, the nucleus is lost.

fatty acid one of a group of organic compounds, each consisting of a long, straight hydrocarbon chain and a terminal carboxylic acid (COOH) group. The length of the chain varies from one to nearly thirty carbon atoms, and may be saturated or unsaturated. Some fatty acids can be synthesized within the body, but others, the essential fatty acids, must be obtained from food. Fatty acids have three major roles within the body.

1 They are components of glycolipids (lipids containing carbohydrate) and phospholipids (lipids containing phosphate). These are of major importance in the structure of tissues and organs.

2 Fatty acids are important constituents of triglycerides (lipids that have three fatty acid molecules joined to a glycerol molecule). They are stored in the cytoplasm of many cells and are broken down when required to yield energy. They are the form in which the body stores fat.

3 Derivatives of fatty acids function as hormones and intracellular messengers.

free radicals in general chemical terms, molecules or ions that have unpaired electrons in their structure and which as a result are very reactive indeed.

gene the fundamental unit of genetic material found at a specific location on a chromosome. It is chemically complex and responsible for the transmission of information between older and younger generations. Each gene contributes to a particular trait or characteristic. There are more than 100,000 genes in humans, and gene size varies with the characteristic, e.g. the gene that codes for the hormone insulin is 1,700 base pairs long.

There are several types of gene, depending on their function. Genes are dominant or recessive. A dominant characteristic is one that occurs whenever the gene is present, while the effect of a recessive gene (e.g. a disease) requires that the gene be on both members of the chromosome pair, i.e. it must be homozygous.

genetic code specific information, carried by DNA molecules, that controls the amino acids and their positions in every protein and thus all the proteins synthesized within a cell. Because there are just four nucleotides, a unit of three bases becomes the smallest unit that can produce codes for all 20 amino acids. The transfer of information from gene to protein is based upon three consecutive nucleotides called codons. A change in the genetic code results in an amino acid being inserted incorrectly in a protein, resulting in a mutation.

glucose the most abundant naturally occurring sugar. Glucose is distributed widely in plants and animals and is an important primary energy source, although it is usually converted into polysaccharide carbohydrates, which serve as long-term energy sources. The storage polymers of plants and animals are starch and glycogen respectively. Other polysaccharides of glucose include chitin and cellulose, which have a structural role and also provide strength.

glycogen often called animal starch, a polysaccharide of glucose units which occurs in animal cells (especially the muscle and liver) and acts as a store of energy released upon hydrolysis.

Grave's disease a disorder typified by thyroid gland
overactivity, resulting in an enlargement of the gland
and protruding eyes. It is caused by antibody production and is probably an autoimmune response. Patients
commonly exhibit excess metabolism (because thyroid
hormones control the body's metabolism), nervousness, tremor, hyperactivity, rapid heart rate, an intolerance of heat and breathlessness. Treatment may follow one of three courses: drugs to control the thyroid's
production of hormones; surgery to remove part of
the thyroid; or radioactive iodine therapy.

hormone a chemical substance that is naturally produced
by the body and acts as a messenger. A hormone is
produced by cells or glands in one part of the body
and passes into the bloodstream. When it reaches
another specific site, its 'target organ', it causes a reaction there, modifying the structure or function of cells,
sometimes by causing the release of another hormone.
Hormones are secreted by the endocrine glands.
Examples are the sex hormones, e.g. testosterone,
secreted by the testes, and oestradiol and progesterone, secreted by the ovaries.

immune being protected against an infection by the presence of antibodies specific to the organism concerned.

immunity the way in which the body resists infection
because of the presence of antibodies and white blood
cells. Antibodies are generated in response to the presence of antigens of a disease. There are several types
of immunity: active immunity is when the body

produces antibodies and continues to be able to do so during the course of a disease, whether occurring naturally (also called acquired immunity) or by deliberate stimulation. Passive immunity is short-lived and is provided by the injection of ready-made antibodies from someone who is already immune.

immunization immunity to disease by artificial means. Injection of an antiserum will produce temporary passive immunity, while active immunity is produced by making the body generate its own antibodies. This is done by the use of treated antigens (vaccination or inoculation). Vaccine is used for immunization, and it may be derived from live bacteria, viruses or dead organisms and their products.

immunoglobulins a group of high molecular weight proteins that act as antibodies and are present in serum and secretions. There are five groups, each with different functions.

Immunoglobulin A (Ig A) is the most common and occurs in all secretions of the body. It is the main antibody in the mucous membrane of the intestines, bronchi, saliva and tears. It defends the body against microorganisms by combining with a protein in the mucosa.

Ig D is found in the serum in small amounts but increases during allergic reaction.

Ig E is found primarily in the lungs, skin and mucous membrane cells and is an anaphylactic antibody.

Ig G is synthesized to combat bacteria and viruses in the body.

Ig M or macroglobulin has a very high molecular weight (about five or six times that of the others) and is the first produced by the body when antigens occur. It is also the main antibody in blood group incompatibilities.

immunology the study of immunity, the immune system of the body and all aspects of the body's defence mechanisms.

immunosuppression the use of drugs (immunosuppressives) that affect the body's immune system and lower its resistance to disease. These drugs are used to maintain the survival of the transplanted organs in transplant surgery and to treat autoimmune diseases. The condition may also be produced as a side effect, e.g. after chemotherapy treatment for cancer. In all instances, there is an increased risk of infection.

immunotherapy the largely experimental technique of developing the body's immunity to a disease by administering drugs or gradually increasing doses of the appropriate allergens, thereby modifying the immune response. The most widely studied disease is cancer, where immunotherapy forms an auxiliary treatment to drug therapy.

irritable bowel syndrome a condition caused by abnormal muscular contractions (or increased motility) in the colon, producing effects in the large and small intestines. Symptoms include pain in the abdomen, which changes location, disturbed bowel movements with diarrhoea then normal movements or constipation, heartburn and a bloated feeling caused by wind. The specific cause is unknown and no disease is present. Treatment is limited to relief of anxiety or stress (which may be contributory factors), drug therapy to reduce muscle activity, and careful choice of diet to include a high fibre content.

ketogenesis the normal production of ketones in the body because of metabolism of fats.

ketone body one of several compounds (e.g. acetoacetic acid) produced by the liver as a result of metabolism of fat deposits. These compounds normally provide energy, via ketogenesis, for the body's peripheral tissues. In abnormal conditions, when carbohydrate supply is reduced, ketogenesis produces excess ketone bodies in the blood (ketosis) which may then appear in the urine (ketonuria).

ketonuria the presence of ketone bodies (*see* ketone and ketone body) in the urine as a result of starvation or diabetes mellitus, causing ketogenesis and ketosis.

leucocyte *or* **leukocyte** a white blood cell, so called because it contains no haemoglobin. It also differs from red blood cells in having a nucleus. Leucocytes are formed in the bone marrow, spleen, thymus and lymph nodes. There are three types: granulocytes, comprising 70 per cent of all white blood cells, lymphocytes (25 per cent) and monocytes (5 per cent). Granulocytes help combat bacterial and viral infection and may be involved in allergies. Lymphocytes destroy foreign bodies, either directly or through production of antibodies.

Monocytes ingest bacteria and foreign bodies by the process called phagocytosis (engulfing microorganisms and cell debris to remove them from the body). In disease, immature forms of leucocytes may appear in the blood, ultimately forming both red and white blood cells.

lipids a term for oils, fats, waxes and related products in living tissues. They are esters of fatty acids and form three groups: simple lipids, including fats, oils and waxes; compound lipids, which includes phospholipids; and derived lipids which includes steroids.

liver a very important organ of the body, with many functions critical in regulating metabolic processes. The largest gland in the body, it occupies the top right-hand part of the abdominal cavity and is made up of four lobes. It is fastened to the abdominal wall by ligaments and sits beneath the diaphragm and on the right kidney, large intestine, duodenum and stomach.

There are two blood vessels supplying the liver: the hepatic artery delivers oxygenated blood, while the hepatic portal vein conveys digested food from the stomach. Among its functions, the liver converts excess glucose to glycogen for storage as a food reserve; excess amounts of amino acids are converted to urea for excretion by the kidneys; bile is produced for storage in the gall bladder and lipolysis occurs; and some poisons are broken down (detoxified). Thus the hepatic portal vein has a beneficial effect in carrying blood to the liver rather than it going around the body first.

The liver also synthesizes blood-clotting substances

such as fibrinogen and prothrombin and the anticoagulant heparin; it breaks down red blood cells at the end of their life and processes the haemoglobin for iron, which is stored; vitamin A is synthesized and stored, and it also stores vitamins B_{12}, D, E and K. In the embryo it forms red blood cells. Such is the chemical and biochemical activity of the liver that significant energy is generated, and this organ is a major contributor of heat to the body.

lymph a colourless, watery fluid that surrounds the body tissues and circulates in the lymphatic system. It is derived from blood and is similar to plasma, comprising 95 per cent water with protein, sugar, salts and lymphocytes. The lymph is circulated by muscular action, passing through the lymph nodes, which act as filters, and eventually returning to the blood via the thoracic duct (one of the two main vessels of the lymphatic system).

lymphatic system *or* **lymphatics** the network of vessels, valves, nodes, etc, that carry lymph from the tissues to the bloodstream and help maintain the internal fluid environment of the body. Lymph drains into capillaries and larger vessels, passing through nodes and eventually into two large vessels (the thoracic duct and right lymphatic duct), which return it to the bloodstream by means of the innominate veins.

lymph nodes small oval structures that occur at various points in the lymphatics. They are found grouped in several parts of the body, including the neck, groin and armpit. Their main functions are to remove foreign particles and produce lymphocytes, important in the immune response.

lymphocyte a type of white blood cell produced in the bone marrow and also present in the spleen, thymus gland and lymph nodes, which forms a vital component of the immune system. There are two types: B-cells and T-cells. B-cells produce antibodies and search out and bind with particular antigens. T-cells circulate through the thymus gland where they differentiate. When they contact an antigen, large numbers of T-cells are generated which secrete chemical compounds to assist the B cells in destroying foreign bodies, e.g. bacteria.

measles an extremely infectious disease of children caused by a virus and characterized by the presence of a rash. It occurs in epidemics every two or three years. After an incubation period of 10–15 days, the initial symptoms are those of a cold, with coughing, sneezing and high fever. It is at this stage that the disease is most infectious and spreads from one child to another in airborne droplets before measles has been diagnosed. This is the main factor responsible for the epidemic nature of the disease. Small red spots with a white centre (known as Koplik spots) may appear in the mouth on the inside of the cheeks. Then a characteristic rash develops on the skin, spreading from behind the ears and across the face and also affecting other areas. The small red spots may be grouped together in patches, and the child's fever is usually at its height while these are developing. The spots and fever gradually decline and no marks are left on the skin, most children making a good recovery. However, complications can occur, particularly pneumonia and middle ear infections, which can result in deafness. A vaccine is now available that has reduced the incidence and severity of measles in the United Kingdom.

menopause *or* **climacteric** the time in a woman's life when the ovaries no longer release an egg cell every month. Menstruation ceases and the woman is normally no longer able to bear a child. The age at which the menopause occurs is usually between 45 to 55. The menopause may be marked by a gradual decline in menstruation or in its frequency, or it may cease abruptly. There is a disturbance in the balance of sex hormones and this causes a number of physical symptoms including palpitations, hot flushes, sweats, vaginal dryness, loss of libido and depression. In the long term, there is a gradual loss of bone (osteoporosis) in postmenopausal women, which leads to greater risk of fractures, especially of the femur. All these symptoms are relieved by hormone replacement therapy, involving oestrogen and progesterone, which is now generally recognized to be of great benefit.

metabolism the sum of all the physical and chemical changes within cells and tissues that maintain life and growth. The breakdown processes that occur are known as catabolic (catabolism), and those that build materials up are called anabolic (anabolism). The term may also be applied to describe one particular set of changes, e.g. protein metabolism. Basal metabolism is the minimum amount of energy required to maintain the body's vital processes, e.g. heartbeat and respiration, and is usually assessed by means of various measurements taken while a person is at rest.

Micro-organism *or* **microbe** an organism that can be seen only with a microscope. Included are bacteria, viruses, protozoans, some algae and fungi.

monocyte the largest type of white blood cell (leucocyte) found in the blood and lymph. It has a kidney-shaped nucleus and ingests foreign bodies such as bacteria and tissue particles.

mucosa another term for mucous membrane.

mucous membrane a moist membrane that lines many tubes and cavities within the body and is lubricated with mucus. The structure of a mucous membrane varies according to its site. They are found, for example, lining the mouth, respiratory, urinary and digestive tracts. Each has a surface epithelium, a layer containing various cells and glands that secrete mucus.

oestradiol the major female sex hormone. It is produced by the ovary and is responsible for development of the breasts, sexual characteristics and premenstrual uterine changes.

oestrogen one of a group of steroid hormones secreted mainly by the ovaries and, to a lesser extent, by the adrenal cortex and placenta. (The testes also produce small amounts.) Oestrogens control the female secondary sexual characteristics, i.e. enlargement of the breasts, change in the profile of the pelvic girdle, pubic hair growth and deposition of body fat. High levels are produced at ovulation and, with progesterone, they regulate the female reproductive cycle.

Naturally occurring oestrogens include oestradiol, oestriol and oestrone. Synthetic varieties are used in the contraceptive pill and to treat gynaecological disorders.

osteoarthritis a form of arthritis involving joint cartilage with accompanying changes in the associated bone. It usually involves the loss of cartilage and the development of osteophytes at the bone margins. The function of the joint (most often the thumb, knee and hip) is affected and it becomes painful. The condition may be caused by overuse and affects those past middle age. It also may complicate other joint diseases. Treatment usually involves administering analgesics, possibly anti-inflammatory drugs and the use of corrective or replacement surgery.

osteoporosis a loss of bone tissue because of its being resorbed, resulting in bones that become brittle and likely to fracture. It is common in menopausal women and can also be a result of long-term steroid therapy.

oxidation any chemical or biochemical reaction that is characterized by the gain of oxygen or the loss of electrons from the reactant. Oxidation can occur in the absence of oxygen, as a molecule is also said to be *oxidized* if it loses a hydrogen atom.

oxidizing agent any substance that will gain electrons

during a chemical reaction. Oxidizing agents will readily cause the oxidation of other atoms, molecules or
compounds, depending on the strength of the oxidizing agent and the reactivity of the other substance.

pancreas a gland with both endocrine and exocrine functions. It is located between the duodenum and spleen,
behind the stomach, and is about 15 cm long. There
are two types of cells producing secretions. The acini
produce pancreatic juice that goes to the intestine via a
system of ducts. This contains an alkaline mixture of
salt and enzymes – trypsin and chymotrypsin to digest
proteins, amylase to break down starch and lipase to
aid digestion of fats. The second cell types are in the
islets of langerhans. These produce two hormones,
insulin and glucagon, secreted directly into the blood
for control of sugar levels (*see also* diabetes mellitus,
hypoglycaemia and hyperglycaemia).

pH the measure of concentration of hydrogen ions in an
aqueous solution. The scale of pH ranges from 1.0
(highly acidic), with decreasing acidity until pH 7.0 (neutral) and then increasing alkalinity to 14 (highly alkaline).

phagocytosis *see* leucocyte.

poliomyelitis *or* **infantile paralysis** an infectious disease caused by a virus that attacks the central nervous
system. The virus is taken in by mouth, passes through
the digestive system and is excreted with the faeces.
The hands may be contaminated, leading to further
spread. The incubation period is 7 to 12 days, and
there are several types of condition, depending on the

severity of the attack. In some cases the symptoms resemble a stomach upset or influenza; in others there is, in addition, some stiffness of muscles. Paralytic poliomyelitis is less common, resulting in muscle weakness and paralysis, while the most serious cases involve breathing, when the diaphragm and related muscles are affected (bulbar poliomyelitis).

Immunization is highly effective, and the disease has almost been eradicated in most countries. However, booster doses are advisable when visiting countries with a high incidence of the disease.

polyuria the passing of a larger than normal quantity of urine, which is also usually pale in colour. It may be the result merely of a large fluid intake or to a condition such as diabetes or a kidney disorder.

protein a large group of organic compounds containing carbon, hydrogen, oxygen, sulphur and nitrogen, with individual molecules built up of amino acids in long polypeptide chains. Globular protein includes enzymes, antibodies, carrier proteins (e.g. haemoglobin and some hormones. Fibrous proteins have elasticity and strength and are found in muscle, connective tissue and also chromosomes.

Proteins are vital to the body and are synthesized from their constituent amino acids, which are obtained from digestion of dietary protein.

proton a particle that carries a positive charge and is found in the nucleus of every atom. As an atom is electrically neutral, the number of protons equals the number of negatively charged electrons. The number of protons in the nucleus of an atom is identical for any one element.

psoriasis a chronic skin disease the cause of which is unknown and for which the treatment is palliative. The affected skin appears as itchy, scaly red areas, starting usually around the elbows and knees. It often runs in families and may be associated with anxiety, commencing usually in childhood or adolescence. Treatment involves the use of ointments and creams with some drugs and vitamin A.

rheumatoid arthritis the second most common form of joint disease, after osteoarthritis, that usually affects the feet, ankles, fingers and wrists. The condition is diagnosed by means of X-rays, which show a typical pattern of changes around the inflamed joints, known as rheumatoid erosions. At first there is swelling of the joint and inflammation of the synovial membrane (the membranous sac that surrounds the joint), followed by erosion and loss of cartilage and bone. In addition, a blood test reveals the presence of serum rheumatoid factor antibody, which is characteristic of this condition. The condition varies greatly in its degree of severity, but at its worst can be progressive and seriously disabling. In other people, after an initial active phase, there may be a long period of remission.

A number of different drugs are used to treat the disease, including analgesics and anti-inflammatory agents.

scarlet fever an infectious disease, mainly of childhood, caused by the bacterium *Streptococcus*. Symptoms appear after a few days and include sickness, sore throat, fever and a scarlet rash that may be widespread. Antibiotics are effective and also prevent any complications, e.g. inflammation of the kidneys.

smallpox a highly infectious viral disease that has been eradicated. Infection results, after about two weeks, in a high fever, head and body aches and vomiting. Eventually red spots appear, which change to water and then pus-filled vesicles that on drying out leave scars. The person stays infectious until all scabs are shed. Fever often returns, with delirium, and although recovery is usual, complications often ensue, e.g. pneumonia. The last naturally occurring case was in 1977.

synovial fluid *see* synovial membrane.

synovial membrane *or* **synovium** the inner membrane of a capsule that encloses a joint that moves freely. It secretes into the joint a thick lubricating fluid (synovial fluid), which may build up after injury to cause pain.

T-cell a type of white blood cell (lymphocyte) that differentiates in a gland called the thymus, situated in the thorax. There are a whole variety of T-cells involved in the recognition of a specific foreign body (antigen), and they are particularly important in combating viral infections and destroying bacteria.

trypsin an important enzyme involved in the digestion of proteins. Its inactive precursor, trypsinogen, is secreted by the pancreas and converted to trypsin in the duodenum by the action of another enzyme called enteropeptidase.

vaccination the production of immunity to a disease by inoculation with a vaccine or a specially prepared material that stimulates the production of antibodies. It was used initially to refer only to cowpox virus (which also protected against smallpox) but now is synonymous with inoculation in immunizing against disease.

vaccine a modified preparation of a bacterium or virus that is no longer dangerous but will stimulate development of antibodies and therefore confer immunity against actual infection with the disease. Other vaccines consist of specific toxins (e.g. tetanus) or dead bacteria (e.g. cholera and typhoid). Live but weakened organisms are used against smallpox and tuberculosis.

virus the smallest microbe that is completely parasitic because it is only capable of replication within the cells of its host. Viruses infect animals, plants and micro-organisms. Viruses are classified according to their nucleic acids and can contain double or single-stranded DNA or RNA. In an infection, the virus binds to the host cells and then penetrates to release the viral DNA or RNA, which controls the cell's metabolism. It then replicates itself and forms new viruses. Viruses cause many diseases, including influenza (single-stranded RNA), herpes (double-stranded DNA), Aids (a retrovirus, single-stranded RNA) and also mumps, chickenpox and polio.